ATTENTION AND FOCUS IN DANCE

ENHANCING POWER, PRECISION, AND ARTISTRY

Clare Guss-West, MA

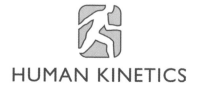

HUMAN KINETICS

Library of Congress Cataloging-in-Publication Data

Names: Guss-West, Clare, 1960- author.
Title: Attention and focus in dance : enhancing power, precision, and
  artistry / Clare Guss-West.
Description: Champaign, IL : Human Kinetics, Inc., [2021] | Includes
  bibliographical references and index.
Identifiers: LCCN 2020023930 (print) | LCCN 2020023931 (ebook) | ISBN
  9781492594451 (paperback) | ISBN 9781492594468 (epub) | ISBN
  9781492594475 (pdf)
Subjects: LCSH: Dance--Psychological aspects. | Dance--Physiological
  aspects.
Classification: LCC GV1588.5 .G86 2021 (print) | LCC GV1588.5 (ebook) |
  DDC 792.801/9--dc23
LC record available at https://lccn.loc.gov/2020023930
LC ebook record available at https://lccn.loc.gov/2020023931

ISBN: 978-1-4925-9445-1 (print)

The web addresses cited in this text were current as of June 2020, unless otherwise noted.

Acquisitions Editor: Bethany J. Bentley; **Managing Editor:** Derek Campbell; **Copyeditor:** Annette Pierce; **Indexer:** Andrea Hepner; **Permissions Manager:** Dalene Reeder; **Graphic Designer:** Joe Buck; **Cover Designer:** Keri Evans; **Cover Design Specialist:** Susan Rothermel Allen; **Photograph (cover):** © Eeva Suorlahti; **Photographs (interior):** © Eeva Suorlahti; **Photo Production Manager:** Jason Allen; **Senior Art Manager:** Kelly Hendren; **Illustrations:** © Lea Bischoff, unless otherwise noted; illustrations on pp. 6, 17, 34, 53, 79, 86, 104, 137, 151, and 192 © Human Kinetics; **Printer:** Versa Press

Printed in the United States of America

10 9 8 7 6 5 4 3 2 1

The paper in this book is certified under a sustainable forestry program.

Human Kinetics
1607 N. Market Street
Champaign, IL 61820
USA

United States and International
Website: **US.HumanKinetics.com**
Email: info@hkusa.com
Phone: 1-800-747-4457

Canada
Website: **Canada.HumanKinetics.com**
Email: info@hkcanada.com

E7982

Tell us what you think!
Human Kinetics would love to hear what we
can do to improve the customer experience.
Use this QR code to take our brief survey.

*To my mother for her courage, faith and light;
to my father for his scientific mind, down-to-
earth pragmatism and humour; and to David,
mon amour, for his unconditional belief and
patience and for sharing this life journey.*

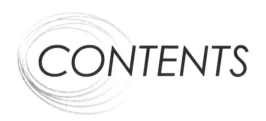

CONTENTS

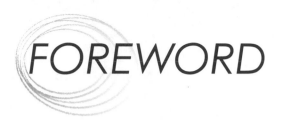

FOREWORD

AN EXTERNAL FOCUS OF ATTENTION IS KEY TO OPTIMAL PERFORMANCE AND LEARNING

GABRIELE WULF, PHD

Movement is a product of the events and processes of the mind, brain, and body, as well as a reflection of diverse influences, from the physical, social, and cultural environment to the body's structure and function.

Rebecca Lewthwaite and Gabriele Wulf (2010)

People are fascinated by dance for many reasons. Among its appeal is the enjoyment of watching or performing skilled, seemingly effortless or aesthetically pleasing movements. The elegance of dance performances is enjoyable from both an observer and performer perspective, and yet we are all aware that the effort typically involved in achieving such highly skilled movement is considerable. A frequently asked question then is whether such extreme physical and mental effort is a necessary component of high-level performance, or can power, precision and artistry be achieved more efficiently and effectively by adopting another approach?

As research over the past two decades has shown, one precondition for efficient and effective motor performance is an optimal focus of attention. I first gained this insight while I was practicing a windsurfing maneuver called a *jibe*: My jibes were unsuccessful when I focused on my body movements, such as my foot position on the board or hand positioning on the boom. In contrast, when I concentrated on my overall movement goal, such as turning the surfboard in a certain direction, I was much more successful. Not only did I manage to complete the jibes more often, but I also did so with considerably less mental and physical effort. Many experienced performers can relate to the consequences of consciously focusing on their body movements, an *internal focus* of attention, instead of a focus on the intended effects of their movements, or an *external focus*. As a researcher, I had the advantage of being able to examine experimentally whether the effects of changing my focus of attention were real and generalizable.

In the first attentional focus study we conducted in my lab (Wulf, Höß and Prinz 1998), we used two different balance tasks. In one experiment, participants were asked to learn a ski-simulator task. While doing so, one group of participants was instructed to focus externally on the pressure they were exerting on the wheels just beneath the platform they were standing on, and the other group was instructed to focus internally on the pressure they were exerting with their feet. A control group received no focus instruction. As it turned out, learning was clearly facilitated by an external focus, compared with both the internal focus and control groups. Similarly, in the second experiment, participants learned to balance on an unstable platform on which two dots had been placed just in front of their feet. Asking participants to concentrate on keeping the two dots horizontal (external focus) as opposed to asking them to keep their *feet* horizontal (internal focus) again resulted in more effective learning.

Since then, the attentional focus effect has been replicated almost 200 times (for reviews, see Wulf 2013; Wulf and Lewthwaite 2016). It is now clear that adopting an external focus of attention is essential for optimal performance and learning. When performers concentrate on the intended movement effect, such as the trajectory of a movement, the movement pathway, the pressure exerted against the ground, the water or the motion of a prop, or even if they are asked to focus on an item of practice clothes rather than on their own body, their movements are more accurate, fluid, effortless, powerful and automatic. In addition, the form of the movement has been shown to benefit from an external focus. These advantages are seen in both immediate motor performance and longer-term learning, and they are independent of the type of motor skill, skill level, age, ability or disability.

When performers think about their body movements, they tend to use conscious control processes that are relatively slow and interfere with more automatic, fast, reflexive control mechanisms. A focus on the self, such as an internal focus on the body, is associated with activation of the brain's default mode networks and has frequently been shown to be detrimental to performance. In contrast, when performers adopt an external focus, they use automatic, unconscious, fast and reflexive control processes that are critical for precise, smooth and fluid actions. An external focus has a dual advantage: It clearly directs attention to the task goal and reduces a focus on the self (or another off-task activity). An external focus likely enhances functional connectivity of task-relevant brain areas, thereby optimizing movement coordination. It is an important contributor to *goal–action coupling*, or the fluidity with which movement goals are translated into actions (Wulf and Lewthwaite 2016). The result is greater movement precision and balance, more efficient muscle activation, reduced heart rate and oxygen consumption, as well as greater sustainability of submaximal forces and greater maximum force production.

These findings have important implications for dance. An external focus facilitates balance performance and results in greater jump height or longer jumps, such as those frequently performed in dance. The benefit of an external focus is especially pronounced when the skills are complex. Moreover, an external focus has been found to enhance the performance in situations that involve pressure (e.g., presence of an audience, competitions). The greater automaticity associated with an external focus has the additional advantage of reducing physical and attentional demands. Thus, performers have more attentional capacity available that allows them to focus on other aspects of performance such as artistic interpretation, musical listening and the actions of dance partners.

In this book, Clare Guss-West describes how she integrates these scientific findings into daily dance practice, education and training. Based on her extensive complementary knowledge and experience of Eastern movement practice and holistic health, she naturally used instructional strategies and techniques that promote an external focus of attention in dance training long before she became aware of the research findings. Translating the human movement science findings with great creativity and ingenuity, Clare uses language, images and metaphors that promote an external focus specifically appropriate to a dance context. By focusing on a chosen image, a dancer's attention is directed away from body movements and onto the intended effect or outcome of the action. Clare successfully applies this approach in her work with professional dance companies and with teachers and therapists, working with a broad spectrum of dance that includes professional dancers, children, older adults and those teaching groups who have movement challenges.

Clare's approach differs from more traditional approaches, some of which are still based on what economist Paul Krugman refers to as 'zombie ideas' (Krugman 2020, para. 4), which are ideas that refuse to die despite overwhelming empirical evidence to the contrary. Examples are that the acquisition and refinement of complex skills make it necessary to focus on body movements, novices need to focus internally, elite performers must benefit from an internal focus, people with a compromised motor system need to consciously control their movements, and simply that dance is different from other movement skills and requires an internal focus. None of these beliefs are supported by experimental findings. Rather they are based on anecdotes or case studies showing that performers improve with an internal focus. Of course, they do – just not optimally!

Teachers, coaches and dancers themselves might become aware of the strength of the evidence favoring external attentional focus and develop an understanding of strategies to identify and maintain performers' externally directed attention. These changes may require creativity and experimentation initially in finding the right external focus as well as include modifications to those foci as a performer's skill level increases. But the benefits are arguably among the most reliable ones available to support effective performance and learning.

In addition to a performer's focus of attention, motivational factors play an important role as well when it comes to successful movement production. Specifically, performer confidence (or enhanced expectancies) and autonomy are critical for optimal performance and learning. Numerous studies have demonstrated the importance of each of these factors. In the OPTIMAL theory (optimizing performance through intrinsic motivation and attention for learning) of motor learning (Wulf and Lewthwaite 2016), all three factors are assumed to make unique contributions to goal–action coupling, to the translation of the desired goal into the actual movement. Indeed, studies have shown that conditions that enhance learners' expectancies (e.g., positive feedback, liberal definitions of success) grant them a certain degree of autonomy (e.g., opportunities for choice, noncontrolling instructional language) *and* promote an external focus and result in even more effective performance than do conditions that involve only one or two of these factors. Clare introduces these additional motivational variables in chapter 7 and looks at their potential application, in combination with an external focus of attention, in a dance context.

Clare Guss-West is at the forefront of attention and focus strategies for dance teaching and performance enhancement. In this book, she shares her vast knowledge and experience as a performer, choreographer, teacher and therapist and provides invaluable suggestions and recommendations that practitioners can use not only to improve dance performance and learning but also to enhance the joy that results from dancing with power, precision and artistry.

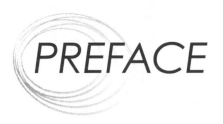

PREFACE

The world behind our eye is our new frontier.

Caroline Myss (2017)

If you could access a kind of inner switch with a simple on–off action in which a small shift of attention produces a synaptic rerouting, unlocking your power and stamina reserves, enabling fluid, efficient movement, heightening your sensory perception and releasing your dancing potential, wouldn't you grasp the opportunity to experience it? Have you reached a plateau in your training and can't progress beyond? Are you losing energy working with so much effort and feeling depleted? This book invites you to find that inner switch, to create the small shift of attention, by bringing your *attention* to the skills of attention and focus. Together we explore this new frontier and discover a systematic approach to the inner work of dance. You'll find a panoply of potent complementary attentional techniques to choose from to enhance physical and artistic performance, to refocus the mind, to replenish energy and to open the pathway to your potential dancing best.

In the last few decades human movement science and sports science have made enormous advances in understanding the role of the mind and the attention and focus in enhancing physical performance. These findings have begun to infiltrate elite sports training – giving the edge to elite performers and their performance.

This exciting body of attentional focus research is at the intersection of Eastern and Western movement practice. Mindful Eastern movement practices such as tai chi, chi kung and kung fu concur with recent scientific findings that a small shift in attentional focus and learning how to filter and guide the attention strategically are key to optimal performance. Such a small shift of attention has the potential to promote an immediate and significant impact on power, precision, balance, consistency, fluidity, artistry and speed of learning and mastery (Wulf 2013, 99).

Given the physical demands of dance, Western training typically prioritizes physical mastery and control of technique over mindful attention. A recent study of professional dancers highlighted that many dancers are experiencing information overload and overthinking their dance in an attempt to consciously control individual body parts during movement (Guss-West and Wulf 2016, 27). A clear lack of a systematic training in mental attention and focus is apparent. This is the training of the inner skills of dance that would further enhance and liberate movement and give dancers the edge in their performance. Science and traditional Eastern wisdom agree that emphasizing physical and muscular control in the absence of a foundation of attention and focus training means that performers are working inefficiently. Many dancers potentially deploy excessive energy and significant counterproductive effort that can lead to global movement dysfunction, lack of stamina, exhaustion and increased risk of injury. Attentional focus training is perhaps then *the* most relevant study that sports science and Eastern movement practice can bring to dance.

Rooted in the 20 years of attentional focus findings of researcher Dr Gabriele Wulf, *Attention and Focus in Dance* is a practical how-to book that introduces a diverse range of attentional focus techniques for dancers, teachers and dance health care practitioners. It aims to act as a bridge connecting research, movement theory and actual day-to-day dance practice. Recent scientific findings are presented and brought to life with direct dance practice and performance and teaching examples. They are illustrated with the beautiful photography of Finnish artist Eeva Suorlahti and the inspirational line drawings of Swiss artist Lea Bischoff, which provide a visual resource that captures the attention, intention and energy in motion. Fresh attentional focus perspectives come from the colourful voices of international neuroscientists, psychiatrists and performance psychologists and also from dancers, teachers and artistic directors who work intuitively with attention to attention in their own practice.

Attention and Focus in Dance is about the *process* of that shift in attention and the *how* of the inner work of dance: *how* we can filter information, *how* we can direct our focus, *how* we are learning, *how* we are teaching and *how* we can cue for optimum physical effect. Developing attention and focus strategies in dance does not require us to forsake or reevaluate our specialist knowledge, our priorities or our expertise, which makes up the content, or the *what,* of our dance: *what* inspires us, *what* we want to prioritize, *what* we teach. Whether technical or artistic, individual specialism is simply rendered more effective by refining the process, the *how*, or the way we deliver it.

Creatively connecting the parallel threads between Eastern movement practice and scientific research enhances performance outcome and learning in diverse contexts. It reflects my own teaching practice in which I draw on this body of ancient and contemporary knowledge to address a range of today's movement challenges, whether minimizing effort and refining movement with professional dancers or enabling movement for all dancing publics.

The foundations of Eastern movement are in complete harmony with many Western dance forms. The parallels are so close that we might imagine that Eastern movement practice actually inspired the birth of Western dance principles. Eastern movement approaches provide additional substance and depth to research data to provide a holistic approach to training, integrating attention and focus techniques that harnesses the power of the breath and the management of energy in motion. The different approaches of these distant disciplines to the same universal movement challenges, with their different language and imagery, speak to different learners and provide alternative inspiration for dance educators.

The evidence-based research findings referred to in this book have been published and referenced in the human movement science literature. The complementary Eastern concepts are presented from the perspective of extensive practitioner experience or practitioner wisdom to provide a fresh approach to universal movement challenges. The ideas presented are developed in a dance-centric format that can be easily adopted and are intended to be used in *existing* training and teaching practice, in rehearsal or in rehabilitation contexts to provide palpable, immediate and long-term benefits to performance results.

> . . . professional dancers are attracted to the simplicity of the systematic application of an *'external'* focus and to the global nature of the benefits experienced . . . [it] promotes an immediate, palpable global movement cohesion in professional, beginners and elderly dancers alike. (Wulf 2015, 1296)

The foundations are laid out in the foreword, contributed by Dr Gabriele Wulf, a distinguished professor at the University of Nevada, Las Vegas, who provides an overview of the body of attentional focus research findings. Attentional focus is positioned in a broader context with other holistic, motivational teaching elements to form the OPTIMAL theory (optimizing performance through intrinsic motivation and attention for learning) of motor learning, and we discover through her work that a holistic approach not only is respectful of the performer but also can be proven to produce measurable, hard-fact benefits to performance enhancement.

Part I, Shifting Attention, is aimed at dancers and begins by looking at attentional challenges and the information overload that many professional dancers currently experience. We review the need for a systematic attention and focus strategy and how scientific attentional focus research relates to dance practice, translating focus theory into dance vocabulary with illustrative focus examples. Chapter 3 takes a look at foundational Eastern movement principles and where they intersect and complement scientific findings, drawing together the threads that unite them. In chapter 4 we revisit with fresh eyes and with this fresh material basic dance elements such as posture, turnout and port de bras to see how these Eastern and scientific concepts can breathe new life into the foundations to renew their sense and their substance. Eastern practice additionally provides dance with inspirational attention and focus techniques for developing stamina, power, speed and precision, and we then integrate them into specific dance challenges such as the sustained, fluid power of the adage, the dynamic balance of the pirouette and the explosive power of jumps and allegro. Part I concludes with attention and focus techniques that performers can use to replenish energy in motion and to protect against energy depletion and exhaustion.

Part II, Cueing Attention, presents attention and focus strategies for teaching, self-coaching and optimal cueing. It addresses frequently asked questions about attentional focus cues for beginners for initial learning of skills and breaking down movements and also for the subtle refining of movement detail for more advanced dancers and professionals. These are supported by practical dance examples and suggestions for implementation in context.

Chapter 7 places attentional focus into a broader context of complementary holistic teaching strategies. We explore aspects such as *how* we are habitually teaching, our choice of vocabulary and how we might support the autonomy of the dancer by giving choices and enhancing expectations. These holistic elements form part of Dr Wulf's larger OPTIMAL theory of motor learning. These additional elements, when combined with attention to attentional focus, are shown to bring further incremental benefits to learning and physical and

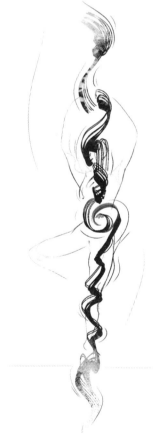

Attention to energy flow to enhance vertical power.

artistic performance (Wulf and Lewthwaite 2016). Part II concludes with a practical guide to optimum cueing, both self-cueing and teacher cueing, and feedback. Cueing for high performance is an art. We explore the question 'If less is more, how much information is too much?' and discover how to format cues and feedback to facilitate effective neuromuscular response and enhance dancer recall of information and accessibility whilst dancing. Cumulatively, these complementary elements empower the performer (Chua, Wulf and Lewthwaite 2018). They enable and align the performers' attentional focus and equip them for the multidimensional demands of the discipline: to produce powerful efficient movement at the service of an artistic objective and intention.

Each of us is deeply individual, the result of our individual experiences, and our paths of learning differ (Watson 2017); therefore, *Attention and Focus in Dance* presents a smorgasbord of concepts and ideas to choose from that have the potential to incrementally enhance learning and performance. I trust you can find food for thought and practical tools for professional and personal expansion within these pages. Take what resonates and what works for you and start to experiment in practice. Leave the rest and perhaps revisit it later at another moment in your dancing journey. The complementary scientific and Eastern elements work cumulatively, so the more ideas and strategies you can incorporate into your daily practice, the more effective they will be.

Be patient. Shifting attention in dance is for most of us like learning a new language: It becomes familiar with practice. Even just becoming aware of where you place your attention, of your distractions, of how you split your focus or talk to yourself whilst you dance is already half of the journey. Use the book as a starting point, an inspiration and a guide to empower you to draw on your own rich artistry, creativity, expertise and experience to develop relevant and personalized adaptations and imagery according to your dance context.

ACKNOWLEDGEMENTS

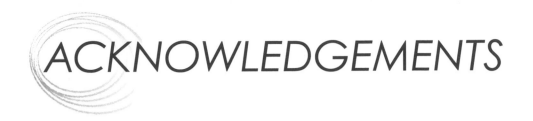

A special thank you to . . .

Finnish National Ballet and artistic director, Madeleine Onne, and senior physiotherapist, Johanna Osmala, for their consistent support of my work;

Dancer Kailey Kaba for her passion and quest and the beautiful dancers Ben Kuefler, Emmi Pennanen and Tehri Talo for sharing their joy;

Artist and photographer Eeva Suorlahti for her sensitivity to capture intention and detail;

Artist and dancer Lea Bischoff for daring to envision the universal and unite the worlds of dance and energy;

Friends and colleagues Raymond Chai, Sorella Englund, Christopher Hampson, Timo Kokkonen, Agnès Lopez Rio, Dr Andrew McWilliams, Dr Sanna Nordin-Bates, Dr Hanna Poikonen, Javier Torres, Stephanie Saland and Dr Gay Watson for taking the time to reflect on their attention and focus in practice and sharing their experiences so generously;

Dr Gabriele Wulf for her inspirational, meticulous dedication to clarifying the attentional process in movement and for her generosity and support of my interpretation in dance;

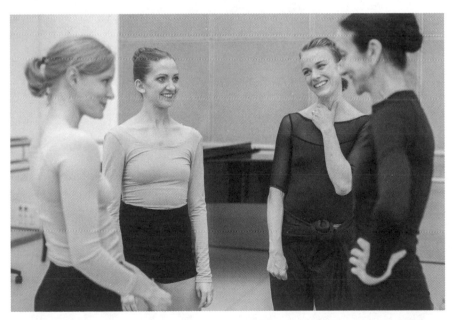

The beautiful dancers of Finnish National Ballet. (Emmi, Kailey and Tehri with Clare)

Greg Retter for his professional support and recognition of the attentional challenges of dancers;

Bethany Lifeso, RAD Canada, and Patti Ashby, RAD USA, for their belief and diffusion of this essential body of work for the next generation of teachers.

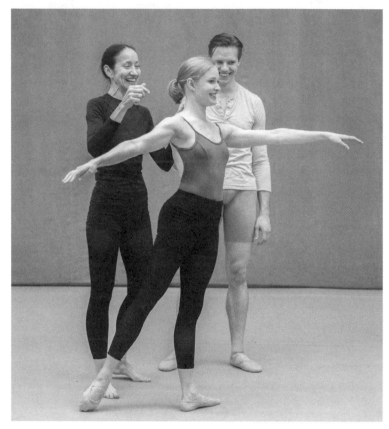

Joy is the essential ingredient in the alchemy of dance. (Clare, Emmi and Ben)

PART I

SHIFTING
ATTENTION

CHAPTER 1

ATTENTIONAL FOCUS CHALLENGES OF DANCERS

The art of being wise is the art of knowing what to overlook.

William James (1890)

*D*ance is perhaps one of the most complex sensorimotor activities that people engage in. It stimulates the maximum adjacent areas of brain function, enhances new synaptic connections and promotes cognitive reserve at all ages. This is essential for full mental and physical well-being (Powers 2010). Dance involves simultaneous cognitive and multisensory, multidimensional perceptual, and attentional demands. These demands include the following:

- An awareness of one's own body movements and the coordination and mastery of the body's moving component parts in relation to one another
- A kinaesthetic sense and an inner proprioceptive awareness of that movement and, at the same time, having the metaskill to visualize its external effect
- An awareness and orientation of the moving self within the space
- A capacity for mental recall of hours of choreographic material (Solway 2007)
- A honed sensory perception to spatially navigate and coordinate that choreography with a partner or group of other dancers, all within the demands of a musical time constraint
- A musical sensitivity and the integration of imagery to enhance a visceral response to stimuli
- A maturing artistic expression and the skills to intentionally transmit and communicate that expression simultaneously to an external audience

These simultaneous demands require enormous amounts of brain plasticity and cognitive reserve. At a professional level today, a dancer – at The Royal Ballet in London, for example – could be performing and recalling as many as three full-length choreographic works on stage at any one time and simultaneously learning and rehearsing up to three other works in the studio, all with different choreographic styles and artistic demands (Retter 2016). In-the-moment demands of performance at a professional level require even more available cognitive reserve to manage additional multitasking and performance stressors such as the following:

- The need for heightened musical listening when working with live musicians and orchestra and therefore potential variable tempi
- Unpredictable objects such as props, unruly costumes and challenging footwear
- A changing environment of designer sets and floor surfaces – perhaps even raked stages

- Extreme onstage lighting conditions different from those used in preparation and training, in which peak performance must be delivered in the dark or in blinding lights, taking away sight as a foundational orientation
- Psychological stressors such as constantly changing team relationships and roles

In addition to the in-the-moment demands of a professional performance, dancers might also be required to recall technical and artistic feedback from teachers, choreographers and rehearsal directors; to access performance enhancement feedback from physical trainers; or to remember remedial or injury advice from the multiple disciplines of a health care team whilst performing. This can cause many dancers, according to Greg Retter, former clinical director of The Royal Ballet, to experience information overload (Retter 2019) (see figure 1.1).

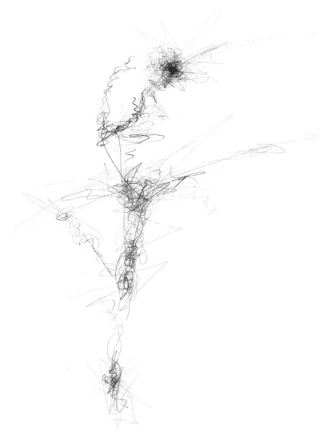

Figure 1.1   Imaginary representation of dancer's attentional fragmentation and information overload.

INFORMATION OVERLOAD

A dancer's journey is far from a dancer-centric journey: A dancer receives professional information from multiple disciplines in each discipline's own specific language. Christopher Hampson, artistic director of Scottish Ballet, confirms witnessing this information overload when dancers receive not only in-house artistic and clinical information but also information from a stream of guest choreographers, designers and dramaturges, who all come with their own specialist languages. At Scottish Ballet they are aware of these information challenges, and the whole team comes together to coordinate any strategic communication to ensure that they use consistent language (Hampson 2019). In most companies, however, it is the dancer's responsibility and challenge to filter all the diverse information. The dancer alone, for the most part, has to manage their own attentional focus demands and decide how they use this diverse information. They must determine how they will process it and make it accessible and relevant to the demands of artistic performance and decide what to filter and what to overlook in the pursuit of optimum performance results (figure 1.2).

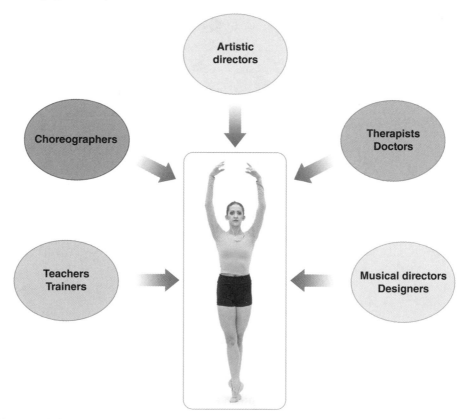

Figure 1.2   A dancer's journey – information overload from the different disciplines.

Added to the professional information is the enormous amount of distracting and distorted information available on the Internet. This fragments dancers' focus and attention further from essential daily preparation and restorative rest, according to former professional dancer Susan Jaffe. 'Wasting time comparing yourself to Insta stars', she suggests, only adds to today's dancer's anxiety and leads to feelings of inadequacy when performance is about the attention and focus to something so much deeper (Thomson 2018, para. 12).

Attention and Focus in Practice

ATTENTION SPLITTING

Dr Hanna Poikonen, neuroscientist, dance educator, dancer

We have seven large neural networks, which we can imagine like highways that connect different regions of the brain. Each network, such as reward, executive control and sensorimotor, has its specific purpose. Some of the networks support the function of others, but the default mode network – the network of mind wandering and emotional introspection – is active only when the activity of the other networks goes down. Basically, the large networks cannot all be active at the same time. Attempts to multitask require different kinds of attentions: One task perhaps requires one neural network, and then another task may need another neural network, and these shifts don't happen so fast. It would be challenging or almost impossible for these neural networks to stay functioning at their optimal level.

More specifically, the default mode network activates not when we are actively involved in a cognitive task or thinking but rather when we guide the attention onto our sensations or our emotions. The default state demands a certain calmness. You cannot be in this mode if you are too alert. When you first practice a complex movement, for example, it stimulates alertness and activates the motor cortex, but once you really know the movement by heart, once it's in the body, the activity of the motor cortex is reduced. So then there is more room for this kind of relaxed state. If we are very stressed or anxious or cognitively overloaded or if someone in the dance class is very focused on the cognitive aspects of the movement, then he shuts down this internal listening and external listening to others. Spontaneity, flexibility and adaptability are also impaired.

There is a kind of multitasking, called multidomain training, in which the tasks support one another, and the functioning of the neural networks is enhanced. However, today when we describe multitasking with a short time span and constant interruptions, harmful attention splitting occurs, which burdens the brain and significantly lowers the quality of the performance tasks at hand.

In a Swedish study to develop sensory awareness and imagery in advanced ballet training, students complained of already having 'too much to think about' in class to be able to focus on learning additional skills, even though these skills were designed to lighten their cognitive load, promote their use of sensory perception and enhance possibilities for artistic expression (Karin and Nordin-Bates 2019).

The conscious effort of trying to attend to all this diverse and sometimes conflicting information and feedback *and* address the actual in-the-moment demands of performance is vying for cognitive 'hard drive' space and undermining a dancer's ability to focus. Without targeted mental training and a systematic attention and focus strategy in place to help dancers wisely filter and cope with these demands, this fragmentation quickly exhausts and blocks available cognitive reserve. *More* is definitely not *more* when it concerns the pursuit of physical excellence. Trying to consciously implement diverse body-related feedback simultaneously in dance dissipates power and effectiveness, undermining rather than enhancing performance capacity (Wulf 2013).

Consider that as dancers, we have undertaken between 10 and 15 years of formative training before we reach a professional level. We have potentially amassed an assortment of formative feedback from diverse sources: notably from early teachers; perhaps also from examiners, competition coaches and judges; and also well-meaning family, friends and perhaps even local general practitioners. We have been immersed in our own cultural environment with its distinctive approach to discipline, effort, achievement, autonomy, freedom and exploration. As British choreographer Wayne McGregor observes, 'in Paris, the dancers have a different physical literacy and history from the dancers here [in the UK] or in Australia' (Mackrell 2009, para. 13). We become the physical embodiment of our early years of accumulative input.

> What we attend to shapes who we become . . . the ability of neuronal processes to be formed and transformed by our attention, shows this to be true . . . the wiring of the brain has been tuned by earlier experience. (Watson n.d., para. 20)

We *are* what we attend to, therefore, and what we choose to remember. The stronger the emotion associated with a memory, the stronger and more vivid the recall from whatever era of our autobiography. Memories that are laid down and embedded with emotions have the quickest neural pathways, making them the most readily accessible today (Jäncke n.d.). Recall of information or feedback whilst under pressure in performance is not necessarily chronological, therefore. It won't necessarily be the most recent technical or health care feedback we were given that comes to mind first whilst dancing. It's most likely to be some of the oldest feedback from formative years that springs to mind under pressure. Until we develop and train our attention and focus, and teachers and coaches implement a systematic attentional focus strategy that renders their feedback accessible during performance, images of princes, swans and frogs from our early training will prevail. Early critical feedback or basic body-part control instructions surface too, sometimes despite our best efforts because they are the most accessible when deeply embedded with emotional cement (see table 1.1).

DEFINING FOCUS AND ATTENTION IN A DANCE CONTEXT

The word *focus* on its own is typically used to describe the act of concentrating and centring the mind, placing attention on a single stimulus (M.S. 2013). **Attention**, however, is much more than concentrating on a single stimulus; it is perhaps best thought of as the process of attending to something (Watson 2017). It involves the process of filtering through the potential surrounding stimuli in any given moment – whether external, internal, present, past or future trains of thought – and deliberately attending only to those that support the demands of the task at hand. It requires, therefore, the ability to consciously defocus from the multitude of other stimuli vying for our attention.

Attention and Focus in Practice

ATTENTIONAL RESOURCES

Dr Andrew McWilliams, psychiatrist, neuroscientist, dancer

Attention is one of the cognitive functions of the mind, and cognitive control of attention is a necessary healthy brain function. Attention is made up of several components: We must be able to identify stimuli of interest, then maintain our attention on the chosen stimuli, monitor our attention and decide when to switch our attention. From a psychological perspective, what a person attends to tells us about who they are. From an artistic perspective, stating our attention to ourselves is a way of saying what's important and getting that across. When there are too many cognitive demands, it's useful for us to have strategies to off-load some of the demands and to manipulate the attentional focus to allow us to have different foci at different times. From a neuroscientific perspective, some processes require more attention from us than others. It's necessary to have an appropriate allocation of attentional resources in order to serve the task at hand. An inappropriate attentional focus would, therefore, not serve our desired ends.

EXPLORATION 1.1 – ATTENTIONAL POSSIBILITIES

Just pause for a moment with the book in your hands and notice how many other stimuli you have been filtering out just now in order to selectively attend to the words on the page and their meaning. Open your ears a moment and focus on the different sounds you can hear. Notice the seat you are sitting on and feel the contact and the pressure. Feel the surface of the floor under your feet. Notice any tension or holding that there might be in your body at this moment. Look up from the book and notice all the different colours of the objects around you. Become aware of the thoughts going through your mind at this moment – perhaps thoughts of things that need to be attended to or a comment of your inner critic. Lastly, just become aware of the flow of your breathing.

So many attentional possibilities are present in every living and dancing moment. How do you know what to overlook, what stimuli to wisely filter out so that your attentional choices support your best performance?

We have several ways to consciously attend to a task or action (Study.com n.d.). We may practice developing a *sustained attention*, which is the process of attending in an undivided way to one stimulus for prolonged periods to the exclusion of all other stimuli. This is the kind of process we use when deeply immersed in a project like planning our choreography and listening repeatedly and attentively to sections of music. We at times use our attention selectively when we need to attend to one stimulus whilst having to consciously block out a lot of other stimuli and distractions. *Selective attention* is operating when we try to listen to a conversation or get feedback in a noisy environment, such as onstage when the orchestra is warming up. We can alternate our attention as we move back and forth between different kinds of stimuli or tasks that require different cognitive functions. *Alternating attention* is operating when we learn movement from a video – for example, we move between focusing on observing chunks of movement material on the screen, and then we attend to the kinaesthetic task of translating that onto our own body. The most common process we use as dancers in training, rehearsal and performance is *divided attention*, sometimes known as multitasking because the process involves attempting to attend to two or more stimuli simultaneously in any one moment.

According to performance psychologist Patrick Cohn, we need to become aware that we are always focused on something and that some foci help our performance while others distract us from performing our best (Cohn 2019). **Attentional focus** then is our ability to sustain a strategy in which the focus of attention is self-guided onto appropriate foci and imagery or guided by a teacher's or coach's feedback cues and instructions (Wulf and Prinz 2001). At the same time as we learn to sustain our focus of attention, we develop our ability to actively filter out all other irrelevant information and feedback, environmental stimuli and streams of thought.

Today, we are aware of the use of mental training in high-level sports and its make-or-break role in the results of performers. Mental skills that increase attention and focus, strengthen in-the-moment attentional ability, and develop resilience against disabling, distracting thoughts are mindful skills that represent a new frontier in elite sports performance. It is the mental skills and attentional focus strategy that high-level performers use that assure their consistent performance and create the possibility for winning genius. More technique training, more conscious control or more strength alone cannot deliver these optimum conditions.

Let's take an example of where mental training might come in to play in a dance context: If, in a dance performance, your first pirouette of a series finishes badly, you might begin to wonder whether you will be able to complete the whole series and secure the variation. Critical thoughts from your early years about always being useless at pirouetting surface. A vicious cycle of distracting thoughts ensues with each subsequent mistake, and anxiety and self-talk increase. In an attempt to keep from losing it completely, you start to pay attention to the basic mechanics of your movement, implementing several pieces of technical feedback that you can recall in the moment to attempt to control the actions of individual body parts. As a consequence, you use more muscular effort and experience a kind of freezing or movement dysfunction that exacerbates the downward spiral and the ability to get back on track (Wulf 2007). Does this sound familiar? In high-level sports, the mental skills to mitigate such a downward spiral, to clear self-talk and to reset the mind, to access enabling rehearsed cues, to stay present in the moment are trained as part of a systematic attentional performance strategy.

Attention, focus and mindfulness training are foundational elements of Eastern movement practice and, as a dance teacher, choreographer and Eastern-movement practitioner, I was already drawing on these fundamentals to support the demands of Western dance training; however, it was only when I began to explore the research findings of Gabriele Wulf that I realized the significant difference evidence-based attentional focus training could make in the development of winning athletes. I began to ask myself about the experience of other dancers. How did they manage the information overload? How did they manage their attentional focus in training and performance?

PROFESSIONAL DANCERS' ATTENTIONAL FOCUS SURVEY

Gabriele Wulf and I started with a study of classical ballet dancers because there seemed to be little literature available on the attentional process of classical training and performance (Guss-West and Wulf 2016). Awareness of the use of attention and focus and mental imagery is more prevalent in contemporary and modern dance forms, whereas attentional strategies are relatively uncharted territory in classical ballet. We developed a simple survey to determine what the typical current focus choices of professional classical dancers were. How did they self-cue to enhance their performance? I wanted to corroborate some of my own direct practical experience as a teacher and choreographer with dancers' attention and focus. The survey addressed both current and former professional dancers. A professional was defined as someone performing full time in a professional company.

We invited the subjects to fill out a short online survey. Participating were 53 current and former professional dancers from 10 countries. Countries included Canada, China, Finland, France, the United Kingdom and the United States to capture a wide range of potential cultural variations in attention and focus. The survey consisted of questions relating to four traditional ballet movements: 'What do you focus on, imagine or think when preparing and executing . . .' A balance in fifth? A balance in arabesque? A pirouette en dehors? And a grand jeté en avant? The movements were chosen in function of their increasing complexity.

The established universality of the classical ballet technique, which transcends cultural boundaries, was an advantage for the survey. It was accepted by the research ethics committee that all professional ballet dancers, no matter their culture, would understand the actions implicit in these traditional movements and would imagine the execution of the same movement based on the given ballet terminology. Dancers were also given the option to participate anonymously. This revealed the personal, almost intimate, nature of a dancer's choice of focus of attention. Nearly half of the participants chose not to reveal their identity in their responses.

We collected over 200 focus descriptions of the four traditional movements. Wulf observed that professional dancers' focus cues showed a high degree of creativity and diversity compared to the cueing she typically observes. My attention was drawn to the fact that for the most part, cues involved large amounts of information and used extensive word formats in comparison to what I had seen of typical attentional focus cueing in sports. If you superficially compare some examples of the attentional focus cues of experienced swimmers that follow with some example responses from the professional dancers' attentional focus survey (table 1.1), what are your immediate observations?

Here are some examples of experienced swimmers' attentional focus self-cues (Stoate and Wulf 2011):

- Getting to the other side
- Pulling fast, fast arms, keep kicking
- Nothing
- Hip rotation
- Speed
- Spinning my arms

- Tempo and pulling lots of water
- Opponent
- Catching at front, pulling hands back

TABLE 1.1   Sample Responses From the Professional Dancers' Attentional Focus Survey

INTERNAL	COMBINATION	EXTERNAL
BALANCE IN FIFTH (DEMI-POINTE OR POINTE)		
Two legs equally balanced through the feet, growing through, back muscles are well engaged, relaxed and well-supported spine through the head.	The pressure of the legs into one another as if they were one or glued and spiraling in opposition.	A sense of energy in two directions: down into the floor and internally lifting up in an opposing direction.
Balancing bones and wrapping muscles.	Ideally a spiral upwards instead of a static, frozen position, with the two legs spiraling outwards from each other.	Reacting to the floor in a crossed-chain sensation, imagining the least resistance.
Core engagement and engagement of muscles of pelvic floor, oppositional forces through the spine, strong fifth position at top of legs.	Pulling up without tucking, arms in front of shoulder, chin lifted, thinking of floating rather than pushing down into the floor.	I imagine elevating myself like a balloon.
BALANCE IN ARABESQUE (DEMI-POINTE OR POINTE)		
I imagine the two arms elongated, the malleolus points to the ceiling, the arabesque leg moves away from the body.	A lengthened curve, the upper body traveling forwards through space whilst the gesture leg curves away from the centre.	Energy expanding out in all directions.
Divide the body in two halves (spine in the middle and both sides) to be able to get a correct alignment of the arabesque, supporting leg is growing through and also into the floor (like in yoga), working leg is lengthened away from the hip joint, arms and neck are relaxed and placed.	I imagine dancing on a big stage and dancing with a lovely partner or doing the balance on the top of the Tour Eiffel, focused on stretching my knees, proper placement, soft arms. I usually hope for a great balance.	Going forward, feeling like a swan.
Foot muscles and straight leg.	Feeling my centre controlled over my supporting leg, the big toe of my arabesque floating away and up, both pushing into and lifting out of the floor as the movement expands.	I imagine stretching like a star in all directions.

(continued)

TABLE 1.1   *(continued)*

INTERNAL	COMBINATION	EXTERNAL
PIROUETTE EN DEHORS		
Relaxing, pushing the knee around and turning with the back.	High on the standing leg, fast to the position.	On a whirligig.
Putting more weight into the supporting leg in plié preparation, keeping width through shoulders, using forward arm first in take-off, then feeling the opposite side of back in conjunction with passé knee and supporting gluteal (muscle).	Complete eye focus, pinpoint spot on floor, carriage of arms, the end of the turn.	Climbing up a corkscrew.
Rotation from hip socket; squared-off hips; coordination of head, back and arms in take-off; use of the floor and appropriate amount of torque.	Just going, too much thinking doesn't help. Keep the body square.	Spiral.
GRAND JETÉ EN AVANT		
Focus is on short foot and gluteal engagement of the push-off leg for thrust, plié accentuated as the ignition.	In preparation going down into the floor for push into the air, imagining staying in the air for two counts whilst pushing legs up higher.	Travelling, achieving airtime in the jeté, gliding through air.
Knees in correct alignment when landing.	Keeping heel down on plié, allowing the music to help find the pause in the air.	I imagine jumping over something.
Releasing the air from my lungs to prevent the shoulders from going up, turning the head to the public.	Jump over a puddle, suspension, soar and glide, with pelvic initiation at top of jump.	On jumping above the lake.

Reprinted by permission from C. Guss-West and G. Wulf, "Attentional Focus in Classical Ballet: A Survey of Professional Dancers," *Journal of Dance Medicine & Science* 20, no. 1 (2016): 23-29.

Many dancers in the study adopted complex, multi-focus or split-focus cues, and there were examples of diverse and potentially conflicting feedback being applied simultaneously to cue the same movement. As an overall first impression, the format of the responses suggested a general absence of any specific, systematic approach to focus, attention and cueing in dancers' training and coaching, despite the professional level of the dancers in the study.

Wulf categorized the study responses into the two established motor learning definitions: **internal** focus of attention and **external** focus of attention. Responses are classified as having an internal focus if they use a clear, self-related focus that refers to the control of a body part or body-part movement such as *knees* in correct alignment, prevent the *shoulders* from going up, working *leg* is lengthened away from the *hip joint*. External focus is determined when responses describe the intended movement outcome or the effect of the movement, and they frequently involve the use of imagery or sensations without reference to the control of a body part or body-part movement. Here are examples – A sense of energy in two directions: down into the floor and internally lifting in an opposing direction. I imagine elevating myself like a balloon. Gliding through air. Another example was simply, Spiral.

In my direct experience of teaching dancers, I have learned that we frequently use multiple types of feedback from diverse sources involving both self-related, conscious body-part control instructions (internal) and mental imagery that focuses on the movement outcome, quality and effect (external) in the same cue. For this reason, Wulf and I identified a mixed category called **combination**, in which dancers clearly combine internal and external foci simultaneously as their chosen control approach. The following are examples: Jump over a puddle, suspension, soar and glide, with *pelvic initiation* at top of jump. Feel the pressure of the *legs* into one another as if they were one or glued and spiraling in opposition. Lift – lightness – fly – stretching *legs and feet*. In research terms, these are still technically categorized as **internal** because, despite the partial external element of the cue (lift – lightness – fly), attentional focus research suggests that the internal, self-related focus (stretching *legs and feet*) cancels out any physical benefits brought by the application of the external focus.

I was interested not only in the content of the dancers' self-cues but also in the formulation and construction of the cueing. *How* were they cueing themselves for optimum effectiveness? Were cues short, clear and concise? Did they have a single focus or multi-focus? Did they mix potentially conflicting information? Were they negatively or positively formulated? Did they use controlling language or supportive language? What vocabulary choices did they use that enabled or inadvertently disabled movement? Could a systematic attention and focus strategy be adopted in dance training to further enhance learning and performance as in elite sports and Eastern movement practices? We will explore further the potential content of attentional focus cues in different movement challenges for maximum physical and mental performance benefits in part I of this book, Shifting Attention. We will address how to improve the structuring and adapting of focus cues and teaching feedback for optimal effect in part II, Cueing Attention.

In the survey of the four traditional dance movements, more than two-thirds of the responses involved a self-related, conscious body-part control focus (internal or combination), suggesting that in the absence of systematic attentional focus training, professional ballet dancers, for the most part, concentrate on trying to consciously control and adjust their own body movements whilst in motion. Nearly a third of the participants, however, spontaneously used external focus of attention cues, perhaps arriving at this control strategy intuitively through personal performance experience or having trained with a teacher who intuitively used external focus of attention feedback cues and imagery to enhance performance.

These findings are in line with studies of athletes who have not received attentional focus instructions or training (Porter, Wu and Partridge 2010). The findings perhaps suggest that in the absence of specific training, it's a human tendency to be tempted to consciously control our own body movements, particularly when the task concerns a public performance that is focused on the correct form of the movement with high expectations of perfect results (Wulf 2013).

Further tendencies in a dancer's changing attention and focus choices were discernable in the study (figure 1.3). Despite the demands of ballet for perfect form and alignment, not all dancers chose self-related, conscious control of the body as their strategy *all* of the time. Their uninstructed focus choices varied depending on the nature and the demands of the movement task itself. They appeared to make different control strategy choices based on the amount of thinking time the movement permitted or possibly based on their perceived difficulty of the task. A balance in arabesque, which is a complex, static balance with a specific desired aesthetic line sustained over a relatively long time, provoked nearly 80 per cent of the study dancers to adopt self-related, internal body-part focus cues. The arabesque also incited the greatest volume of self-cueing material. Given the aesthetic concerns for correct line and the sustained duration of the arabesque, it is perhaps only natural, in the absence of specific attention training, that dancers are tempted to interfere and to consciously try to control their own limbs and body parts. It seems that the more time there is available to think or worry about the result, the more dancers choose self-cues to try to manage or adjust the arabesque.

In contrast to the arabesque, a balance in fifth position – a simple static balance with a less challenging aesthetic line – did not incite the use of one particular focus strategy for managing the task. Dancers perhaps perceived less difficulty and, therefore, used a variety of foci drawn from their previous training or personal preference. They also used noticeably fewer words to achieve this balance.

A pirouette en dehors – a combination of a dynamic balance with rotation and demands for a precise form and controlled closing – typically provokes increased performance stress in many dancers. Perhaps as a result of anticipating perceived difficulty and the resulting increase in stress, the dancers in the study proposed the greatest number of combination cues, the combination of internal body-part control and an external attentional focus strategy on the desired effect of the movement. To conquer pirouette anxiety, are dancers enticed to use all possible focus feedback at their disposal simultaneously in performance? The choice of combination cues created split-focus demands for the dancers that further challenged attentional ability.

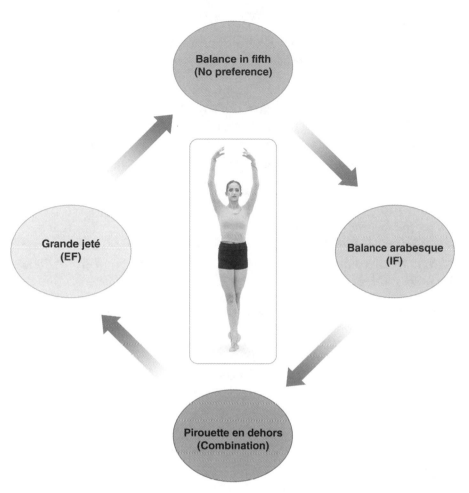

Figure 1.3   Without attentional focus training, different tasks provoke the spontaneous use of different kinds of foci (Guss-West and Wulf 2016, 23-29). EF = external focus; IF = internal focus.

Responses for the grand jeté en avant, on the other hand, were mostly in sharp contrast to the responses for the other tasks. The grand jeté – a dynamic, ballistic action – promoted the most concise, spontaneous use of external attentional focus cues on the desired effect of the movement. Given that the explosive jump leaves little or no time for thinking or conscious control, dancers are obliged to find brief, external focus cues and clear mental imagery to support the desired movement outcome.

Overall, the survey confirmed my own experience: There is, in general, a lack of a systematic attention and focus strategy or of consistent mental training for dancers, in comparison to the heavy emphasis placed on physical training. Mental training would provide much-needed complementary tools to lighten the physical demands of technique and, at the same time, enhance available energy, power and cognitive potential. Moving forwards from the study we might conclude that mindful attention to the process of attention and focus in training and performance will be the next frontier in dance as it has become in elite sports.

> You can approach mental skills in the same way that you approach the physical and technical parts of dance . . . if you consistently work on your mental skills, you will improve them, and your overall performance will benefit. (Taylor and Estanol 2015, 13)

This new frontier beyond physical training is an exciting opportunity for dancers. It promotes autonomy and empowers dancers to develop the skills to adapt and self-manage, enhancing performance resilience. For teachers and coaches, the complementary teaching tools offer the possibility of developing skills that further enhance teaching efficiency, promoting optimal learning and dancers' retention.

> Attention is like a muscle that becomes stronger and more controllable over time. (Watson 2017, 250)

The next chapters explore how a specific attention and focus strategy in movement can bring instant and long-term physical and mental benefits. We will practice easy-to-use examples that can be integrated, as complementary tools, into your regular dance practice for immediate effect. We'll look at how a focus strategy may be introduced into dance education or into a professional dance environment, not only to maximize performance, learning and retention but also to support the well-being of the dancer and provide new skills for a sustainable career.

REFLECTION PROMPTS

Moving to the next level of performing potential means the beginning of a new, exciting journey, awakening your awareness to the processes of your mind as a performer and bringing your attention to the process of your attention. Following are reflective questions to prompt your first steps of this new exploration:

- During exploration 1.1, how many attentional stimuli were you able to identify? So many possibilities are present in every living and dancing moment. Are you aware of filtering stimuli to support your attentional choices? How do you do that?

- Ask yourself the same four questions posed to the dancers in the professional dancers' survey. What do you focus on, imagine or think when preparing and executing a balance in fifth? A balance in arabesque? A pirouette en dehors? A grand jeté en avant? Jot down your spontaneous responses. We will come back to them later and you can choose whether you would consciously change any aspect of your self-cueing.

- Comparing yourself to others, as Susan Jaffe says, only increases feelings of anxiety and inadequacy. Anxiety increasingly shuts down your capacity to perceive, to listen, to respond and to adapt, which are vital for enhanced performance and artistry. With the prevalence of the Internet and the competitive nature of the dance world, what kinds of strategies could you use to support your focus on the deeper, more meaningful elements of dance?

- Did you recognize yourself in some parts of the pirouette discussion: the vicious cycle of conscious control or distracting thoughts? In daily training or other dancing moments when you are not under too much pressure, start to become aware of some of your attentional choices or interrupting self-talk whilst you dance. Just observe for now without judgement.

A reflective journal is a great support tool to accompany you through the practical exercises in this book. Use it to capture inspirational moments as you develop your awareness and develop your attentional focus skills. Enjoy the journey!

CHAPTER

2

ATTENTIONAL FOCUS: A SCIENTIFIC PERSPECTIVE

Attentional focus research is one of the relevant and appropriate bodies of knowledge that sports science can bring to dance.

Greg Retter, former clinical director, The Royal Ballet
(personal communication, 2019)

*A*ttentional focus is an exciting body of kinesiology research. It's the study of *how* we guide our attention in movement, *how* we might optimally cue ourselves to focus or *how* we guide dancers and students to effectively place their attention and concentration whilst learning and refining movement skills. In this chapter we bring our attention to the process of attention and shine a light on our habitual, go-to control processes and ask these questions. How might we modify our current, chosen or unconscious control approach to promote our optimum performance? What are the specific benefits? How might we change the wording of cues to enhance physical and artistic results? How could we start to integrate an attentional focus strategy into our daily dance practice?

The attentional focus findings and practical suggestions here aim to provide complementary tools to explore this new frontier and enable your existing dance practice to evolve to the next level. These complementary tools do not require that you reevaluate the content of your dance practice, the *what*. We will focus only on the *how* – how you currently control and cue your dance. Whatever the particular dance discipline, style, expertise or body of knowledge that you bring to dance, you will be able to grasp these complementary tools and take advantage of the findings and benefits to enhance your performance and effectiveness. I teach attentional focus skills for a wide range of disciplines. I teach professional dancers, dance teachers and teachers of older adults and people with special needs. I also work with multidisciplinary dance health care teams, musicians, singers, conductors, arts educators and health care workers and help them develop effective collaboration and communication skills based on attentional focus research findings. A systematic approach to attentional focus in training is more prevalent in Olympic and high-level professional sports, where it is delivered as essential training to give performers a winning edge. It is relatively new to the dance world. A few professional companies such as Finnish National Ballet, The Royal Ballet and Houston Ballet, and some vocational education organizations such as the Ballet School of the Finnish National Opera and Ballet, Le Pôle National Supérieur de Danse Rosella Hightower, The Rudolf Nureyev Foundation and The Royal Academy of Dance have recognized its potential to transform training approaches and teaching.

At whatever skill level, whether you are working with beginners learning movement skills for the first time, with preprofessionals mastering movement or with professionals refining performance or are working in rehabilitation or with older adult dancers recovering movement skills, developing an attentional focus strategy in your practice brings multiple benefits to facilitate learning and enhance performance results.

ATTENTIONAL FOCUS – DEFINITION

The 20-year body of attentional focus research in movement-skills learning, introduced by Dr Gabriele Wulf in the foreword, confirms that significant differences to the speed of learning and to performance results occur depending on our chosen attentional focus and the chosen wording of our cueing. Research has consistently shown that what kinesiology terms as an ***external focus of attention*** (EF) has significant advantages over what is termed an ***internal focus of attention*** (IF). These terms are not concerned with a performer's *visual* focus, but refer to the guiding of a performer's concentration and attention (table 2.1). A performer may need a *visual* focus out front on the horizon, for example, and yet their attention may be concentrating on the verticality of their movement or on a chosen metaphoric image. The kinesiology terms refer to two different approaches to the placing of the attention or concentration. Both have the same objective – the control and mastery of movement – and both approaches have the same intention to facilitate and enhance performance results. Many examples exist of researchers and educators using the terms imprecisely, which has led to some confusion (Wulf 2013). Therefore, it is important to understand the definitions of these two terms from the outset.

The term *external* is not limited to the external environment, and the term *internal* is not referring to inner sensory information and feedback as one might perhaps guess if taken at face value. Sports coach Greg Dea simplifies the definition of internal attentional focus versus external to a focus on **parts** (IF) versus a focus on **patterns** (EF). An external focus approach highlights

TABLE 2.1   A Description of Internal and External Focus of Attention

AN INTERNAL FOCUS OF ATTENTION	AN EXTERNAL FOCUS OF ATTENTION
Draws the attention to a body part or to body-part movement. This type of cueing or instruction is self-focused. It heightens access to the inhibitive, conscious, self-invoking schema and promotes the conscious control or adjustment of body parts (internal). Instructions are characterized by the naming of the body part or parts.	Guides the attention to focus on the movement outcome, trajectory, pattern, quality or effect. This type of cueing or instruction sustains the attention on the desired movement to facilitate fast, reflexive, automatic movement adjustment (external). Instructions are characterized by their absence of a named body part or parts.
Examples: Instructions such as lower the shoulders, lengthen the neck, open the back, lift the leg, focus on your fingertips, turn the legs out, stretch the foot.	Examples: Instructions such as create space, elongate towards the ceiling, sense the opening, increase the angle, send energy out, spiral down into the rock, sharp accent out.

patterns of movement and overcomes the challenges inherent in trying to consciously coordinate and control many moving parts. In sports, external focus is also referred to as task focused because the performers' attention is guided towards a task that is *outside* of themselves (Dea n.d.).

If we take the example of an expert archer, it is no surprise to most of us that the expert archer adopts an external attentional focus: He is perhaps firmly rooted in the ground, attending to the desired flight path or trajectory of the arrow and clearly concentrating on a distant object or target. We don't imagine for a moment that he is consciously attending to the mechanics of his own body movement, thinking of engaging his core muscles for stability, or that in the moment of peak performance he is instructing himself to lower the shoulder and adjust the hand grip in order to achieve the correct flight path and hit the target. These instructions would logically fragment his attention and undermine his performance. Research confirms that the performance of accomplished professionals may be significantly undermined simply by taking their attention back to self-related foci on the mechanics of a body part or body-part movement (IF) (Wulf 2007). Even small modifications to the wording of instructions or cues can have a significant impact on the effectiveness and efficiency of movement skill performance – small modifications such as the seemingly inconsequential difference between 'press *your feet* into the floor' versus 'press *your shoes* into the floor'. The significant impact on effectiveness and efficiency has been proven for multiple types of human movement skills, regardless of whether the movement involves an external, physical target or not (Wulf 2013).

ATTENTIONAL FOCUS – RESEARCH

The list of confirmed advantages of adopting an external attentional focus approach in learning and performance is extensive (see table 2.2) (Wulf 2013). Perhaps the easiest to perceive initially in dance practice is the direct impact it has on balance, precision, speed and force production, or power. As we shift attention between IF and EF, the effects are immediate and palpable, as if we had accessed a neuromuscular on–off switch or a neural network rerouting. Attentional focus skills are honed with practice; however, it is satisfying for dancer and teacher alike to experience the immediate physical differences as soon as we change the focus of attention:

- Muscular activity is immediately more efficient, and inappropriate effort is reduced, resulting in less fatigue and greater stamina. The heart rate is lowered and oxygen and energy consumption are minimized.

- Movement patterns become visibly more fluid and movement quality more masterful. In human movement science, quality is measured by the number of movement units or visible interruptions to the flow. A

high number of interruptions is typical of novice movement in comparison to the minimal number of movement units used by a professional
dancer in a masterfully smooth, seamless transfer of weight.

• Improved automaticity of movement frees up cognitive reserves to
permit multitasking and attention to in-the-moment performance
demands. It also provides the cognitive freedom to attend to artistic
objectives that require heightened sensory skills such as listening,
perception and emotional interpretation.

The simple shift of focus to an external focus produces these benefits
simultaneously as one global, cohesive, automatic movement adaptation. This
occurs at all skills levels and across all ages. It applies to injury rehabilitation
and stroke recovery and in cases of attention-deficit/hyperactivity disorder
and other attentional disorders and neurodegenerative conditions such as
Parkinson's disease (Wulf 2007).

Over 80 published research papers confirm the benefits of introducing an
EF approach to movement control, so let's take a look at a few examples of
motor skills that are most relevant to dance. Early research involved simple,
single motor skill tasks such as balance or jumping. In a jumping study,
participants were asked to simply jump as high as possible (Wulf and Dufek
2009). They were asked to do this using an internal focus of attention by
concentrating on reaching high with their arm and focusing on the ends of
their fingers (IF). The same participants were then asked to repeat the task,
this time with an external focus of attention and were instructed to reach
high and focus on the measuring equipment (EF). Focusing on their intended
movement objective, on the equipment (EF), the same participants were able
immediately to jump significantly higher than during the IF trial as a result of a
more efficient engagement of muscles and resulting greater force production
or power promoted by the simple shift of focus.

In a more complex coordination, expert swimmers were also asked to use
an IF and an EF for different laps of the crawl stroke. Swimming is much closer
to dance for me, because the desired movement should be powerful and yet
graceful, fluid and economic. Swimmers move alone without obvious external
props or goals, working only with their own body and the surrounding water.
They affect their immediate external element (the water) as dancers do as
they push through the surrounding air. The swimmers were asked to focus
on the action of their hand as they pushed back for their IF laps and to focus
on the movement of the surrounding water as they pushed back for their EF
laps (Freudenheim et al. 2010). To assure the integrity of the research, the IF
and the EF instructions should both describe the same movement objective
and aim to control and enhance the same aspect of the movement. Wording
of IF and EF cues in research is therefore almost identical, with just a minimal
modification to shift the focus. With this simple shift away from the body

action (IF) to focus on the movement of the surrounding water (EF), these already expert swimmers were able to improve their own best speed by using an external focus of attention. This improvement in speed is a global result of the simultaneous benefits of greater fluidity, improved movement quality and economy of movement with more efficient muscular coordination and increased power promoted by the external focus of attention.

Another study that is relevant to dance looked into the ability to sense, recall and implement appropriate effort in movement (Lohse, Sherwood and Healy 2011). In this study, participants were asked to press a measuring plate on the floor with 30 per cent of their maximum force. The plate measured their accuracy and then their ability to recall and accurately replicate the 30 per cent effort in a later trial. The IF instruction required participants to focus on their calf muscle working with 30 per cent of their force, and the EF instruction was to focus on pushing the floor (measuring plate) with 30 per cent of their force. In the EF trials, in which participants focused on the movement objective to press the floor, participants were almost twice as accurate as in the IF trials in which they tried to control their own muscular engagement. In the same study, intermuscular engagement was compared and was found to be significantly increased during IF trials with unnecessary muscular recruitment in the lower leg when participants focused on the control of their calf muscle (IF).

Accuracy and form were then studied in young, training gymnasts who were working on a more complex movement, a half-turn jump with correct landing position (Abdollahipour et al. 2014). For the study, the correctness of the form of the movement was evaluated and deductions made for each error in landing placement. For the IF trials, the gymnasts were asked to focus on the direction their hands would point after their jump. In the EF trials, a sticker was placed on the breast bone and they were asked to focus on the direction the sticker would point after the jump. Immediately, as with other jump research, the EF trials showed a significant increase in jump height; however, the important element was that the EF also resulted in significantly improved *movement form and accuracy*. EF trials showed almost 50 per cent less error in landing placement than the IF trials, confirming that accuracy and the learning of a specific form are greatly enhanced by the use of an external focus of attention.

Other studies have confirmed the immediate, increased cognitive reserve associated with instruction using an EF. Participants in a balance task, as in other simple balance studies, were able to produce faster, automatic microadjustments to maintain their balance whilst using the EF instruction. However, they also demonstrated a heightened attentional capacity to react to a simultaneous secondary task that was given whilst balancing when using the EF instruction. The EF resulted in faster response times than in IF trials, suggesting that participants had free cognitive capacity when using an EF (Wulf, McNevin and Shea 2001).

For dance and for other disciplines that involve more complex movement challenges such as performing music or gymnastics, it's significant that the *more* complex the demands of the discipline, the *more* pronounced are the benefits of adopting an external attentional focus (Wulf, Töllner and Shea 2007). Professional musicians playing a piece of their own choice were rated by experts from the perspective of technical accuracy and artistic expression (Mornell and Wulf 2018). The raters were 'blinded', that is to say they were unaware of the focus instructions given to the musicians. The IF instructions asked musicians to focus on their finger movements and the correct notes, and the EF instructions asked them to focus on the expressive quality of the music and the communication with the audience. The musicians were rated from a technical perspective on several criteria: precision, control, rhythmic stability, clear phrasing, correct dynamics and fluidity. From the point of view of artistic expression, they were rated on the depth of their understanding of the work, the coherence of their artistic gestures, their emotional interpretation and their presence on stage. Focusing on the expressive quality and communication with the audience (EF) understandably produced a pronounced higher rating in terms of artistic expression; however, it also resulted in significantly higher ratings of *technical precision* relative to a focus on the conscious control of the finger movements (IF). In a test, or control, trial in which the musicians were asked to play as they would normally without other instruction, all of them responded that they had focused on the conscious control of their body and finger movements at some point. Research suggests that the slightest, self-related conscious control focus is enough to produce a less-than-optimal performance (Wulf et al. 2010). Even simple self-reflection is shown to interfere with motor skill activation and performance (Jarrett 2015). A performer's tendency to consciously focus on the control of their own movements in performance may be the result of previous IF training instructions, of their own habitual IF control preference or the fact that in the absence of an attentional focus strategy, it's only human to become more self-conscious in public. It's believed that external focus cues reduce the tendency of conscious interference and allow for optimal neuromuscular organization (McNevin, Shea and Wulf 2003). Learning to direct attention towards the music and the expression (EF), as in the study just described, and away from the self is a necessary development to enable an enhanced, masterful, technical and artistic performance (McPherson and Zimmerman 2011).

In addition to the extensive benefits that attentional focus training promotes – lightening and supporting the physical and mental demands of today's dance technique – its use as a systematic feedback and cueing strategy across a whole multidisciplinary team (artistic and teaching staff and health care professionals) provides a cohesive answer to dancer information overload and fragmentation. The act of dancing demands a divided attention (the ability to process two or more responses or process demands simultaneously); however, by implementing as a team a communication strategy based on EF, we free up a dancer's cognitive reserve, allowing the dancer to better attend to these multiple process demands and still have freedom to focus on the artistic objectives of their role.

TABLE 2.2 Proven Benefits of an External Attentional Focus Approach to Movement Learning and Performance

BENEFITS TO MOVEMENT	FOR WHOM
Enhanced learning: • Speed of learning to acquire movement skill and accurate form • Improved recall and long-term learning, permanent changes	• Children and adult beginners learning initial movement skills • Preprofessionals mastering movement skills • Professionals refining movement skills and performance • Older adult learners recovering movement skills • People recovering from injury • People with ADHD and other attentional disorders • People with Parkinson's disease • People recovering from stroke
More effective movement: • Balance – fast microadjustment • Precision • Consistency • Enhanced, appropriate force production or appropriate power	
More efficient movement patterns: • Power – maximized force production • Speed • Fluidity – a global, cohesive movement correction and optimal coordination patterns • Minimized muscular activity • Increased stamina and minimized fatigue as a result of lower heart rate and reduced oxygen and energy consumption	
Improved movement quality	
Increased movement automaticity	
Additional cognitive reserve: • Allows multitasking – fast reaction time • Ability to manage performance stress	
Enhanced artistic interpretation (Mornell and Wulf 2018)	

Based on G. Wulf, "Attentional Focus and Motor Learning: A Review of 15 years." *International Review of Sport and Exercise Psychology* 6 (2013): 77-104.

ATTENTIONAL FOCUS – HOW DOES IT WORK?

Research suggests that adopting an external attentional approach that focuses on the movement effect, pattern or outcome allows the body to use its automatic control processes that are unconscious, fast and reflexive. These automatic control processes produce a much more efficient collaboration of our physical and mental resources than when we attempt to consciously organize our movement. Attempting to control the movement with conscious thought appears to block this reflexive ability for automatic adjustment, resulting in less-than-optimum muscular engagement and coordination, inappropriate force production, excessive energy expenditure and slower inconsistent movements that are easily exhausted. Using a self-related, con-scious control (IF) appears to link what should be semi-independent body parts and thereby diminishes the effectiveness of the motor system. An EF does not promote such constraints but allows the automatic motor system the freedom to microadjust accordingly to achieve the desired movement intention and effect (Wulf 2013).

Professor Rich Masters suggests that consciousness came much later in our evolutionary process and that before we learnt to formulate self-related thought, we used a sophisticated, nonconscious, perceptual function that displayed a variety of advantages in comparison to the later conscious cog-nitive processes, particularly with regards to optimum movement. If when facing a tiger, Masters explains, we were anxious and consciously thinking about our stone-throwing movements and ability (IF), our reaction time and movements would have been too slow and we would simply have been eaten. So evolution meant that only those people using the unconscious perceptual function survived. Masters proposes that we access these vestigial unconscious brain mechanisms by using an external focus of attention (Eightyeightdays 2018; Masters 2014).

Interfering with the body's sophisticated automatic control processes, although no longer a question of life or death, does temporarily paralyse movement, producing what is known as a choking or freezing reaction that spreads far beyond the named or adjusted body part to extend throughout the adjacent muscle chain. Otherwise semi-independent body parts engage to produce a more global movement dysfunction (Zachry 2005). Wulf pro-poses that just the *naming* of a body part in cueing or feedback is enough to invoke the neural representation of the *self*. The *self*-system appears to be easily accessible and easily triggered in all movement contexts, leading to self-related adjustment and self-evaluation, microchoking or freezing and diminished overall performance in movers from beginner to professional alike (Wulf 2013).

Although using neuroscientific research to explain the functioning of this phenomenon is in the early stages, studies of visual imagery ability by Pidgeon and colleagues, for example, suggest that certain neural processes irrelevant to the task are suppressed by using visual imagery (EF) (2016). The amount of intracortical suppression has been shown to positively influence motor performance, and a recent study has shown that switching from IF to EF creates immediate changes to inhibition processes and organization in the primary motor cortex of the brain. The study speculates that the increased inhibition during EF might contribute to the better movement efficiency associated with this attentional focus (Kuhn et al. 2016).

ATTENTIONAL FOCUS IN DANCE

Let's take a look then at what these research findings might mean to us in our day-to-day dance training, how we might benefit from them and begin to apply them effectively in our practice. Let's start with the example of a simple balance in fifth (figure 2.1) and consider it from the perspective of both IF and EF control approaches – how might we instruct a successful balance and perhaps even an artistic suspension. Typical IF instructions for a balance in fifth might be to squeeze the legs together, lift out of the hips and lengthen the neck – for example, a focus on parts. An EF approach to the same movement objectives could be achieved through the instructions to push the floor away and reach through to the ceiling – a focus on trajectory, quality, outcome or patterns. This is merely a matter of semantics you might think; however, the effects are immediate and palpable.

A balance in fifth is not particularly challenging for most dancers, so that makes it a perfect place to start trying the two approaches and clearly identifying the different sensations they elicit. If you are teaching and want to try this in class, divide the class into active dancers and observers because the feedback from the observers is usually as astute and surprising as the self-reported sensations of the active dancers.

EXPLORATION 2.1 – COMPARE AN IF AND AN EF ATTENTIONAL FOCUS CONTROL APPROACH

Let's do a series of balances in fifth, arms in fifth or couronne, progressively stepping forwards. We'll take the series twice: once with IF instructions and once with EF instructions. Take a series of perhaps three or four balances with each focus type so that you can observe and register what's happening in your body. Come down between each balance, take a large step forwards, and refresh the attentional

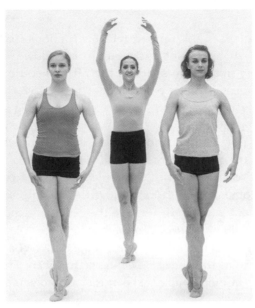

Figure 2.1   Example IF and EF instructions for a balance in fifth –
'squeeze the legs together' (IF) or, as an alternative for the same movement objective, 'push the floor away' (EF). (Tehri, Kailey and Emmi)

focus and balance with the other foot in front. Remember this is not about visual
focus, so perhaps take the eye line out directly in front in both versions. Choose an
appropriate music to accompany the balances if you wish; however, use the same
music both times.

   If we start with the IF version, I ask the class first to shout out typical body-focused
control instructions for a balance in fifth. For this exercise I'm going to suggest three:
legs together, stomach in, shoulders down. Aim to keep your attention on only those
three focus instructions, even if you are normally excellent at balance and have your
own well-established balance cues. If you have observers, ask them to shout out the
three IF instructions as if they were sport coaches, as loud and insistently as they
can. So, off we go . . . up on demi-pointe, arms to fifth and balance . . . legs together
. . . legs together . . . stomach . . . stomach in . . . shoulders down . . . shoulders . . .
legs . . . legs . . . stomach . . . and so on. Aim for 30 seconds in each balance. Come
down, relax and posé (step) forwards with the other foot . . . demi-pointe and . . .
legs together . . . stomach in . . . shoulders down . . . and so on for a series of three
or four balances, and relax.

   How did that feel? What did you feel happening in your body? Were you breathing?
How much effort were you using? Was the balance successful? Did you feel you were
dancing? If you have observers, ask them to describe what it looked like to watch.
Your sensations will be easily accessible when you have just experienced the activity,
so perhaps jot down a couple of key words whilst they are fresh to remind you of
the sensations you experienced when using an internal focus.

(continued)

Now let's take that again, this time with EF instructions. To keep the movement objectives parallel, I suggest using these cues: press down into the floor, reach through to the ceiling, maximum space in the fifth or couronne. Everything else should remain the same. Observers or 'sport coaches' ready? They should be as loud and insistent as the first time around. If you're experimenting alone, keep the three cues clearly in your mind. Repeat and refocus them each time you come down. Off we go. Demi-pointe, port de bras and balance . . . press the floor . . . press down . . . reach through to the ceiling . . . reaching through . . . make space in the fifth . . . maximum space . . . reach through . . . reach . . . press . . . space . . . and so on for about 30 seconds. Coming down, release and posé (step) forwards on the next side and . . . press the floor . . . reach through to the ceiling . . . make space in the fifth . . . and so on for a series of three or four balances.

Did that feel different from the first series? If so, how? What did you feel in your body? Were you breathing this time? How much effort were you using? Did you feel like you were dancing? Could you hear the music? Could you hear the music in the IF series?

Ask the observers to compare the two. What did this look like to watch? Can they identify differences? Again, jot down a couple of key words to remind yourself of the sensations you experienced when using an external focus.

Here is typical feedback I hear when participants use an IF: It was so exhausting. I never breathed. I felt fragmented. I felt so constrained. I wasn't dancing. The typical feedback when using an EF: That was much lighter. I felt free to express. I heard the music for the first time. I was actually dancing. Observers usually give feedback that the IF version was not attractive to watch and used too much effort and tension. For the EF version, their feedback is usually that it looked more expansive; the dancers were bigger somehow; they were whole, calmer, much more constant; and it was more engaging to watch.

This simple balance activity is not trying to establish whether the 20 years of research is correct; it is trying to help you develop your own visceral understanding of the different outcomes and sensations that the two approaches provoke. If you could not identify differences in this first activity, be patient. It might mean that the balance in fifth is not challenging enough for you! Remember, the benefits of using an external focus are more pronounced the more complex and challenging the task.

HOW TO DEVELOP EXTERNAL ATTENTIONAL FOCUS IN DANCE

What types of external foci might we choose from to guide the mind and the attention onto the desired movement outcome, pattern, effect or quality? In sports, EF types can perhaps seem more easily identifiable because there are often more physical, external objects such as balls, rackets, an opponent or a goal to focus on. In dance, external focus options might appear less obvious at first; however, we do have plenty of tangible, physical external elements that we already work naturally with that may be used as potential EF. These tangible elements could be the floor, our clothing or costume, a partner dancer (figure 2.2), the music or the dramatic role. However in dance, we have a huge advantage in that we are already highly skilled and creative at using other more subtle external foci such as proprioceptive and sensory information, qualitative movement dynamics, musical movement dynamics, auditory information, emotional and interpretative information, mental anatomy imagery, mental metaphorical kinaesthetic imagery, mental metaphorical visual imagery and imaginary movement visualization, which are all excellent EF possibilities to choose from (Pavlik and Nordin-Bates 2016). (See figure 2.3 for examples of potential external focus types and table 6.1 for examples of EF types to address different learning styles.)

The EF possibilities in dance are limitless and range from tangible external physical objects and elements related to the movement, to more subtle foci on the movement effect, such as sensory, imaginary or visualized foci. Research findings suggest that the physical and mental benefits promoted are the same whether we choose a real, tangible or imaginary EF (Lohse and Sherwood 2011; Lawrence et al. 2019). So the type of EF you choose will depend on your personal preference or the preference of your dancers. While it might at first appear challenging to shift habitual ways of working and to develop alternative EF cues, you will find that a small adjustment in the focus or to the wording bring immediate benefits. A systematic shift to EF, for example, might be as simple as a return to prioritizing artistic external foci such as the musicality of the movement or the relationship and touch of other performers (see figures 2.2 and 2.3).

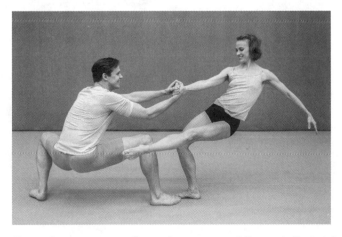

Figure 2.2   Focusing on a partner dancer and the relationship in movement (figure 2.3, number 5). (Ben and Tehri)

Real	Tangible	Sensory	Imaginary
1			20

1. Floor, stage scenery, lighting	11. Sound of the movement against the floor: the brush, the glissé (slide), the chassé (chase), the frappé (strike), the landing, the fall, the teacher's sounding
2. Dance clothes, shoes, costumes, hats, props, masks	12. Touch: the proprioceptive recall of the physical touch of a partner dancer, peer, teacher or therapist
3. Stickers, bands, tape, markers, balls, props and other physical teaching resources	13. The flow of the breath through the movement
4. The movement effect: description of movement directions, form, dynamics, quality: • In, up, out, down, high, close, croisé (crossed), diagonal • Straight, curve, circling, arc, spiral • Accent, attack, suspend, crescendo • Extend, lengthen, resist, press, contract, fly, sharp, fondu (melt), glissé (slide), enveloppé (envelop)	14. Sensing and moving through the surrounding field of oxygen – displacing, interacting with the air
5. A partner dancer or the relationship in movement to other dancers (see figure 2.2)	15. Metaphoric imagery (informing movement form): make a triangle or square, like an elevator, like a barbecue spit, like a tripod, like the Eiffel Tower
6. Choreography	16. Metaphoric imagery (informing movement dynamics): move like melting ice cream, a jellyfish, a lever, scissors, like you're on stilts, on a tightrope, like a tornado, a shooting star, a fountain of water or a wave
7. Touch: the physical touch of a partner dancer's support, a peer, a teacher or therapist's feedback	17. Metaphoric sensory imagery (informing quality and dynamics): move through water, a field of lavender or mud, like sticky honey, squashing marshmallows, working bread dough, chopping cucumbers, pushing the sand or feeling the sun's rays
8. Musical listening for musical colour, rhythm, accents, dynamics, texture, emotion	18. Directing the flow of energy through the movement and beyond
9. Story, dramaturgy, context, role, empathetic response, emotional interpretation of the work	19. Directing imagery, mental rehearsal or 3D visualization of one's own optimum movement pathway in space
10. Proprioceptive recall of having used stickers, props or other physical teaching resources	20. Sensing and moving through the surrounding universal electromagnetic field of energy – displacing, interacting with the flow of energy (see figure 2.4)

Figure 2.3 Examples of potential external focus types in dance on a spectrum ranging from physical, tangible foci (1-10) to sensory and imaginary foci (11-20).

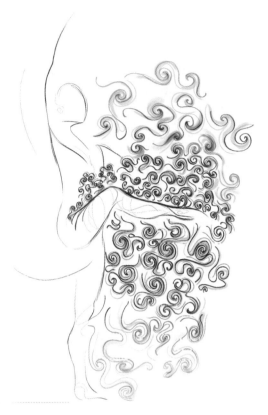

Figure 2.4   Sensing and moving through the surrounding universal electromagnetic field of energy – displacing, interacting with the flow of energy (figure 2.3, number 20).

Benedicte Bemet, senior artist with The Australian Ballet, discusses in the video *Ballet Anatomy: Hands* the importance of touch as a focus in dance.

> Your hands are probably the most important thing in partnering. A lot of the steps rely heavily on how the boy has his hands on your waist. With weight transfers, with turns, with lifts, the pressure with which you hold hands, **touch** is such an important sense which helps you set up a mood and carry that through the piece. (Australian Ballet 2018)

Bemet describes her attention on a partners' touch on her waist (EF) and the importance of all the implicit information that comes through the touch to effect the successful execution of so many technical elements of dance. Attention to the pressure of a hand hold (EF) can inform the intention of a whole choreography.

The spectrum of EF types proposed in figure 2.3 could be used as the basis for a gradual implementation progression. As you start to expand the use of EF in your dance practice, perhaps start with cues and feedback that are more tangible (figure 2.3 1-10), and as you become more fluent at using them, gradually include more sensory – energy flow – imaginary or visualization foci (figure 2.3 11-20). Some dancers have a more naturally developed attentional focus ability than others; however, attentional focus is a skill that can be learnt, just as we learnt physical dance technique. Dancers' ability to use more subtle and complex imagery choice (EF), for example, appears to develop in parallel with technical skills (Pavlik and Nordin-Bates 2016; Nordin and Cumming 2006; Nordin and Cumming 2007).

EXTERNAL ATTENTIONAL FOCUS CONTENT

The actual content of the EF listed in figure 2.3 is of course your choice and will differ enormously from dancer to dancer and teacher to teacher depending on the dance style, skill level, expertise, priorities, culture, gender, age and interests. The possibilities are as infinite as our own creativity. Much has been written about the potential content of metaphorical imagery for dance technique and performance that you can use for inspiration and to develop your own imagery repertoire further (Pavlik and Nordin-Bates 2016; Franklin 1996). No *one* prescribed image, however, works for everyone, so be creative and inventive when searching for inspirational content. Whatever your chosen content, keep in mind that it's *how* you guide attention onto the movement pattern or effect and *how* you format the wording of the content to draw focus away from the *self* that makes it an EF, not the specific content choice itself. So for example, if you use the metaphorical image of wings in a port de bras, you might imagine 'Expand your wings and feel the wind between the tips of the feathers' (EF). However, with the same image, you could also instruct yourself to 'Open your arms like wings and keep the fingers soft' (IF). Follow the EF suggested definition (table 2.1) and aim to cue your chosen imagery so that it focuses you clearly on the objective of the movement and its desired quality, pattern, effect or outcome without naming body parts. Be aware that your chosen wording might inadvertently bring the focus back onto the conscious control of body parts (IF) despite your choice of a beautiful metaphorical image.

An external attentional focus approach is not new to dance. Many professional dancers and inspirational teachers over the years, through the process of practitioner wisdom, have come to understand intuitively the benefits of using external attentional foci. For the most part, however, dancers and teachers tend to use an EF sporadically or spontaneously, when feeling inspired to do so, or just for certain skill types such as a lyrical port de bras or allegro (jumping) or at certain more relaxed times in dance training. Many are unaware that a systematic application of an EF control approach has the potential to transform any aspect of technique, particularly the most demanding and arduous. Often, when the going gets tough or when anxiety rises, precisely when an EF approach would provide the greatest benefits and performance assurance, many dancers and teachers revert to self-related, conscious control feedback, instructions and cues (IF) in a misplaced belief that a return to body part control in challenging circumstances would produce a better result. The less-than-optimal performance results that we so often put down to nerves or stress come frequently from self-determined interference that overrides the body's superior, automatic, regulation processes. The exciting body of attentional focus research, then, validates what many dancers and teachers sense intuitively. It empowers them to continue to use EF with authority as a preferred strategic control approach to enhance the learning of all dance technique and skill types and to promote consistently improved performance results, under all conditions.

EXTERNAL ATTENTIONAL FOCUS – DISTANCE EFFECT

An additional phenomenon has been observed that enhances incrementally the benefits of an EF according to its **distance** (real or imaginary) from the body, or the *self* (McNevin, Shea and Wulf 2003). It appears that the further the focus is guided from the self, the greater the benefits experienced. According to research, there is no particular apparent superior *direction* away from the body for the distal attentional focus, so it could be forwards or backwards, up or down, or in all directions simultaneously. Again, the intuitive use of this phenomenon of a distant focus is not new to dance; many professional dancers and teachers intuitively use a distant focus of attention when they want to enhance a particular movement highpoint or artistic intention in choreography. They use foci such as reach for the stars, explode like a fire-work, or communicate with the audience or focus on *one* instrument in the orchestration to further refine their performance. Rather than systematically introducing the use of distant EF as a strategy, performers typically deploy these types of distal EF spontaneously as well. Dancers and teachers may easily, unwittingly contradict the cohesive, beneficial effects of the distant EF reach for the stars by adding a last-minute IF instruction such as 'and remember to keep the shoulders down' that brings us back to 'earth' to the *self*-evoking schema and undermines all the benefits promoted.

The progressive *distance* in dance parallels to a degree the spectrum from real, tangible EF to sensory and imaginary EF (figure 2.3). A near or proximal EF is often a more tangible, real EF (e.g., floor, shoes, sticker, prop). We might simply choose to move the focus from proximal to distal EF by increasing the physical distance of the attentional focus (e.g., to progress from 'reach through

A JOURNAL OF EXTERNAL FOCUS IDEAS

Kailey Kaba, professional ballet dancer, Finnish National Ballet

In pursuing perfection within my technical form, I would overthink and feel my breath constrained, tense with information overload. Imagining a rond de jambe movement, my brain would fire off a hundred corrections that I would expect my body to respond to and execute immediately. 'Rotate your leg, point your foot, support and hold your arms, widen your back, lengthen your neck.' It's overwhelming thinking in parts. Dancing feels stuck and restrained instead of freeing. Artists are not machines. While we work to be technical and strong, the individual search and exploration in expression is the interesting part for both the viewer and artist. It is a magical moment and then it's gone. When you explore and expand within emotional creativity movement, you have so much more fun and energy to share.

In my Journal, I've collected inspirations and ideas from teachers that have resonated for me:

- Imagine clear energy lines flowing vertically, horizontally, diagonally: It's simpler for my mind to process and allows me to focus on expanding my movements in different directions.

- Paint, sketch and colour your dancing. Maybe one day you play with colour and another day sketch in black and white; don't forget highlights and shadows. Play with the qualities of your movements and paint your own canvas: Vary thickness of stroke, short or long, and add different colours. The canvas is the space around you – the breaths you take, the lines you create and move through with your arms and legs.

- Let the music translate through your body. Use its energy: the fortes and pianissimos.

- Focus on pushing down for strength and stability – not just down through the leg, but continuing through the pointe shoe and the whole line through the crown. Energy doesn't stop where your physical form ends. Your movements need to expand beyond.

I go back to these often depending on the demands of the day. I've learned not to panic if I lose direction; it happens to the best of us. Being open and receptive to new ideas challenges one to grow, think differently and expand. (Kaba 2019) *the shoes'* for a glissé or jeté action to focusing the attention farther away towards a spot or *marker on the floor* or to the *corner of the studio*) to enhance the quality of the movement. However, increasing the *distance* of an EF in dance often involves using a metaphorical or imaginary focus. For example, the proximal, tangible EF instruction 'push the floor away' that we used for the balance in fifth might become something like 'press down to the *ground floor*' or even further away, 'reach down into *the rock*', in order that it becomes more distal. With the action of a prop (EF) – a fan, for example – the attentional focus could progress from 'focus on the circling of the fan' to 'imagine the waves as you displace the surrounding air'. In the same way that we might choose to make progress along the spectrum from a real, tangible EF to a more subtle FF, some dancers might find it easier to begin with the more proximal EF and work towards more distal attentional foci as attentional skills and dance skills develop in order to take advantage of the further incremental benefits this distance provides (see table 2.2 for the benefits of an EF).

IMPLEMENTING AN EXTERNAL ATTENTIONAL FOCUS APPROACH

Deciding to make this systematic adjustment to our attention and to become aware of our cueing language is a relatively small shift compared to the magnitude of the evidence-based physical and mental advantages it has to offer. As with making any change, it requires a conscious commitment to develop our awareness and shift our habitual ways of controlling and cueing movement. The big advantage is that this EF control strategy is complementary to our current dance practice and supports our own dance specialisms and priorities for effective training.

For some dancers and teachers, however, making this shift might prove more challenging than it sounds in theory. Adopting an EF movement control strategy may feel at first like giving up direct, conscious control of the movement and produce the sensation of doing less. Developing an EF approach does not constitute giving up control. Quite the reverse, it's choosing to implement a rigorous, proven, alternative control strategy that guides the attention away from self-evaluative and self-regulating processes (Wulf 2013) to focus clearly on the task and the desired movement effect in order to provoke significant increases in strength, stamina, energy, speed, balance, fluidity and precision (table 2.2). If we have habitually trained to strive for technical excellence by using self-regulating conscious control and are used to the associated sense of having a direct control over our movement, this approach will feel *normal* or as if it were simply *part of who we are*. Changing from our habitual control approach could even be experienced, in some cases, as a personal threat (Karin and Nordin-Bates 2019). Deciding to make the shift of attention in this case may involve initially simply developing awareness of the two control options and trusting that awareness will foster a growing consciousness and gradual loosening of the self-related control option.

Dr Andrew McWilliams, a psychiatrist and dancer, proposes that our habitual control strategy could be regarded almost like a style of positioning our focus and our attention as a dancer. Traditional dance training may promote perfectionist tendencies or might be attractive to those with existing perfectionist tendencies, he reflects. Perfectionism is closely associated with the desire for conscious control.

As one of the participants in a ballet study on perfectionism suggested, 'It felt like technique disappeared a bit . . . it still becomes good, in a different way' (Karin and Nordin-Bates 2019). Using EF, dancing may suddenly seem much freer, take less effort or feel as if you are doing less than usual. I think of dancing with an EF control approach like surfing waves or skiing black runs: High-level performers need a control approach that supports precision in the technical movement form but also supports their heightened reflexive sensory capability so that they can react fast and fluidly in the moment to the demands of the waves or the snow. Similarly, in order to achieve our optimal performance in dance, we need this same state of freed-up cognitive reserve for automatic microadjustments to occur in balances, pirouettes or sustained movements. It also allows heightened sensory capabilities for musical listening, interpretation and artistic expression, and allows us to react to in-the-moment challenges from partner dancers or unknown performance

Attention and Focus in Practice

THE DESIRE FOR CONSCIOUS CONTROL

Dr Andrew McWilliams, psychiatrist, neuroscientist, dancer

It's not necessarily about wanting to be perfect, but rather about wanting to be *sure* you have done your utmost within your capability to achieve the best 'you' that you can be . . . and this is where it interfaces with self-consciousness and control. Some dancers may feel that intense self-control is something to aspire to and they may welcome more and more self-regulating control as a goal. Furthermore, teachers may go on to encourage these tendencies, either inadvertently or on purpose, as they also believe they are desirable. I can imagine it's challenging for some to take a different relationship with their body and allow that to have an effect on their body and to see where that goes. Ultimately, young dancers may be successful, not because of their perfectionism, but rather may be having to learn to achieve in spite of it.

stressors that might arise. If we are thinking or controlling, we simply cannot be present in our dancing. Like the surfer, the dancer needs to be economic with conscious thought processes and with the desire for self-regulation and adjustment because these activities block significant amounts of cognitive capacity. Imagine your brain like your computer: thinking and controlling require large amounts of gigabytes of your 'hard drive', blocking efficient, high-speed intra-(neural) network communication. For mastery and excellence, the dancer must rely on the body's wisdom and allow its fast, reflexive processes to make constant adjustments to efficient muscular engagement, verticality, balance and speed without conscious interference. This ensures the most economic use of resources: of heart rate, oxygen distribution, energy and nutrients for optimum power and stamina. The dancer in the perfectionism study concluded that the creative, imaginary and sensory foci (EF) of the intervention actually promoted 'real' dancing (Karin and Nordin-Bates 2019). However challenging it may appear at first, developing awareness of your habitual control process is the key and enables you to move away from what feels like simply *part of who you are* and make a quantum shift in both your technical skills and artistic capacity to support the best *you* that you can be.

The research findings are particularly robust suggesting that an external focus of attention is the optimum control approach for movement. The process appears to override individual preference. In some studies participants were asked to choose their preferred control process (IF or EF), and then asked to perform a movement task using both their preferred focus and then the other. Despite their personal preference, the EF approach systematically provided enhanced performance results every time (Marchant et al. 2009; Weiss, Reber and Owen 2008; Wulf, Shea and Park 2001). Participants who preferred to consciously control and adjust their own body movements (IF) outperformed their habitual best when shifting their attention to an EF. This means that the attentional focus mechanism itself has a stronger influence on performance outcome than a performer's personal focus preference.

As you decide to introduce EF self-cueing or instruction and feedback into your dance practice, become aware initially of how much of the time you currently focus on and name body parts and use conscious self-correction (IF). Developing awareness of your current, habitual control process is already 50 per cent of the journey towards implementing a change. We know from recent studies that both dancers and athletes when left alone to their own devices without attentional focus training or a specific strategy attempt to consciously control body parts around 70 per cent of the time during training and performance (Porter, Wu and Partridge 2010; Guss-West and Wulf 2016). Looking at that from a positive point of view, that means that they are already intuitively using EF self-cueing around 30 per cent of the time whilst dancing without being particularly aware of the process. Integrating an EF approach into dancing and teaching is not as much of a polarized, black and white, either–or process as research might suggest, but in practice it is rather more likely to be a sliding scale of IF to EF. If you estimate your IF attentional focus use to be within the range documented in the studies, then you are already using EF intuitively in about 30 per cent of your dancing – fantastic! *Any* increase in your use of EF will be a bonus and will provide immediate, palpable benefits. Perhaps give yourself an initial goal of using an EF approach for 50 per cent of your dance practice, which doesn't seem so radical. To put it in perspective, I have been developing my awareness of habitual control strategies and proactively working to integrate an EF approach in my dance training and teaching for over 10 years, and, as a teacher, I am probably operating on average about 90 per cent EF instruction, cueing and feedback in class. This might fluctuate from 75 to 100 per cent EF depending on many variables. I've noticed that I use more IF instruction when I'm teaching online and more EF when teaching live. So, although we can deduce from scientific research that 100 per cent EF is the ideal, this is perhaps an unrealistic 'perfectionist' goal. I suggest that life, art and dance practice is somewhat more 'grey' than that. Start with a goal to develop consciousness around how you currently control your movements, notice how you habitually self-cue or instruct in class, and see any incremental increase in using EF as a first step on the journey towards enabling your heightened dancing power, precision and artistry.

REFLECTION PROMPTS

This chapter about the established scientific findings prompts a lot of reflection. Although the research has been developed over the last decades, the practical application of these fascinating findings lags far behind. The findings provide plenty of new complementary tools and possibilities to choose from that we can begin to integrate creatively to our advantage in our dancing.

Take a moment to jot down a few thoughts about how these scientific findings relate to you and your dance practice. Let's review your current movement control preferences as a starting point for your explorations:

- Do you have an idea of your preferred or habitual movement control approach today? Are you more comfortable consciously controlling the movement form and the body yourself or do you enjoy using qualitative description or imagery to guide the movement effect?

- Do you use both approaches perhaps at different times, like many other dancers? What is the typical ratio of IF to EF you use: 70:30, 50:50 or already something like 40:60? Can you score yourself today? *Note:* When you reflect, you might find that this differs according to the dance context.

- Take a moment to reflect on when you predominantly use each approach whether in self-cueing or teaching. Is it related to the style of dance? To the task (e.g., adage versus jumping)? To the context (e.g., in training, while improvising, while rehearsing, in performance, in exam or competition)? To your mental state (e.g., EF when you're feeling relaxed and confident, and IF when the pressure is on and you're feeling more stress)?
- Look again at figure 2.3 and note how many of the possible EF types you already use when you dance or teach. Give yourself a score out of 20.

Now you have a good idea of your habitual control approach today. We'll come back to your notes later and see whether you score yourself differently and whether habitual choices have shifted in practice.

CHAPTER

3

ATTENTION AND FOCUS: THE INTERSECTION OF EASTERN AND WESTERN MOVEMENT

Think about all those practices . . . of attention and mindfulness . . . of chi kung — all of these practices are about centering your focus . . . that releases something in your body or makes new synaptic links or changes the way you think about the brain/body connection.

Royal Ballet resident choreographer, Wayne McGregor
(quoted in Watson 2017, 241)

The process of attending to attention and focus and the understanding of the ensuing physical and mental benefits are central to many Eastern movement practices and martial arts: Chinese forms such as chi kung and tai chi, Japanese forms such as aikido or Indian yoga practices. The recent attentional focus research findings of human movement and sport science we explored in chapter 2 concur with many elements of the traditional teachings of Eastern movement practice. Both agree that a specific choice of focus and attention can have a significant impact on movement performance: on power, precision, speed, fluidity, balance, economy of movement and stamina. In this chapter we take a look at some of the fundamental principles of attention and focus from an Eastern movement perspective in the movement family of chi kung, tai chi and kung fu and see how these ancient teachings intersect with the recent research findings in human movement science. We explore how an understanding of both of these perspectives can provide valuable complementary tools for dancers.

THE MEETING OF EASTERN AND WESTERN MOVEMENT PRINCIPLES

Chi kung, tai chi and kung fu are related forms that represent a progression of movement in terms of power, speed and complexity. Chi kung, denoting *energy work*, deals with foundations of human movement such as managing energy and breath for movement effectiveness. It focuses on the inner working of the moving body – on developing awareness and attention, on the use of conscious breath, and promoting optimum energy flow and fluid movement for maximum efficiency. Tai chi is based on the same movement forms and foundations but progresses to become *moving energy*, building on these inner foundations to focus additionally on more complex physical movement forms and more diverse movement qualities. Lastly, kung fu, which literally denotes *hard work and training*, uses the same foundations of breath and energy and physical forms. However, it focuses on developing power by turning up the energy volume to become an explosive, fluid, precise movement form that increases speed and develops stamina. The accumulated knowledge of nearly 5,000 years of practitioner wisdom in attention, focus, energy and breath in human movement (Brecher 2001) can be translated to apply to any human movement discipline and has much bearing on the current performance and focus challenges of dancers today. This family of somatic movement practice is particularly appropriate because it shares many of the same demands as dance. It requires an inner awareness and proprioception and yet a simultaneous external awareness of the precise movement form and movement objective. It also requires a mastery of spatial orientation and a relationship to a moving partner. Attention and focus principles refined in these ancient forms complement the performance demands of dance and can be applied directly to dance practice without conflicting with dance objectives and can be used as supplementary tools to enhance physical and mental performance.

My own realization of the potential of this meeting of Eastern and Western movement principles came about as the creative result of a professional dance injury. After more than 25 years of intense Western ballet and contemporary training, professional performing and choreographing, I was injured, exhausted and depleted of vital reserves of energy. I removed myself from the demands of professional dance and retrained in holistic health, rehabilitation massage and, fortuitously, chi kung practice. As dancers do, I launched myself 100 per cent into my new direction, beginning with publishing a book about my mind–body approach to dance recovery, then lectures on mind and self-healing until I became a managing director of an international wellness company. The path of recovery took me far from my roots and my love of dance. Living in Paris, I would walk past the dance studios du Marais every day. Little by little, the music filtering through the windows and the familiar smell of dance infiltrated my being until I realized that despite success, I was actually 'home sick'. I wondered whether I dared go back to class. I summoned my courage to stand at the back of the class of former Béjart Ballet dancer Katalin Csarnoy and to start again from scratch to get to know my new body – to mold muscles and adapt effort to classical ballet demands. To my immense surprise, as well as to that of the colleagues who knew I had not danced or trained for 15 years, I discovered a stronger me. I had more stamina, more jump height, more ballon, more speed and more breath than at 20 years of age. I was dancing with a new lightness and economy and an ease of movement I had never experienced in my professional years. I was fascinated with the question of why an immersion in another discipline could have brought all these qualities unconsciously to my dance. Feeling like a fish back in water and thrilled to have opened another new challenging chapter of dance in my life, this was the burning question: Is this transferable to other dancers?

In an attempt to answer this question, I started a pilot class in Paris. I'm ever thankful to the group of experienced, mature dancers who were willing to experiment with me, a crazy English woman. I integrated chi kung principles of attention, focus, energy and breath into ballet class, with the objective of minimizing effort and maximizing economy of movement to lighten technique and enhance certain performance results. Participants concluded that integrating the new concepts was progressive and as with any new 'language', practice and time were essential factors in becoming fluent. However, some spectacular breakthrough moments were experienced immediately, notably in adage, allegro and pirouette. Participants noted a new ease of movement, improved power, sustain, stability and stamina and reduced performance stress. After six months of once-per-week complementary training, the majority of the dancers in the class said they were able to sustain the new language and integrate the complementary tools effectively in their other regular daily training environments, even in the absence of a supporting or reinforcing teaching voice.

One of the most fundamental differences between an Eastern approach and a Western approach can be witnessed in our relationship with art, according to Dr Gay Watson, a specialist in mind sciences. In the West, she explains, we are primarily concerned with perception and tend to observe art from the outside, to see it as an object. We form opinions of what we *think* about a work and we, therefore, experience it as separate from us (Watson 2017). In the case of the art of dance, this means we focus primarily on what we can see – the form, the line and the positions – how the movement looks. From the dancer's perspective, this leads to a tendency to dance from the *outside in*: explicitly for others such as teachers, artistic directors and spectators. In an Eastern approach, art begins with respiration and is experienced as a process; the focus is placed on how the living work *feels*. The feelings evoked become a shared journey between artist and receiver. An Eastern approach to movement begins, therefore, by developing this inner work of dance: the feel of the movement and the experience of human fundamentals such as the breath and the flow of energy coordinated with simple movement. We clear rather than fill the mind and develop attention skills to enable optimum movement efficiency, power and precision: We work from the *inside out*. This approach might be illustrated by a traditional Chinese saying that suggests we should naturally first learn how to *fill the tea pot before pouring the tea* (Collette 2019).

Another significant difference is the construction of movement itself. The chi kung family of movement is based on a continuous, circular flow of movement and energy throughout the form. The focus priority is on the quality of the connecting movement between two positions and not on the arriving at the position itself. This approach might be likened to the focus and quality of temps liés exercises in ballet that focus on the connecting movements. Although we might imagine that this requires a slow, deliberate transition, in the faster form of the movement family – in kung fu – it is precisely this fundamental mastery of continuous motion that permits speed, precision, fluidity, economy and power. A Western construction of a movement phrase might be seen as a series of curved effort trajectories that use power to initiate a movement until the movement reaches its peak, is exhausted, dies off before gathering energy again to initiate the next movement, and so on. A focus on the continuous, circular flow, however, means that our movement has no point of exhaustion or doesn't die off. In kung fu, a point of exhaustion would be considered a weak point and an opponent would seize the advantage and strike. The concept of continuous circular flow produces an extremely economic, efficient movement and as a result, enhanced, long-duration stamina. Some Eastern practitioners find a typical Western approach to movement – using maximum muscular engagement and effort to sweat and push ourselves until we are spent and exhausted – difficult to comprehend. From an Eastern perspective, this unnecessarily depletes vital energy and is counterproductive because without economy of movement, we won't have sufficient staying power to effectively build strength and stamina.

Despite these differences of approach, the chi kung movement family shares several elements of external form with traditional classical ballet:

- Posture – elongated spine, lengthened occipital bone and neutral pelvis for maximum energy flow to the vital organs
- Port de bras forms – half and full port de bras that gather, lift, give and lower energy through the body; a preparatory breathing port de bras before the start of each form and the bras bas closing and lowering that contains energy at the end of each phrase
- The progressive use of an outward rotation of the legs (turnout) for maximum range of motion
- The use of a systematically deepening plié for increased circulation and power
- The progressive use of demi-pointe for more powerful energy flow through the movement
- Temps liés and detailed actions such as fondu, tendu, rond de jambe and transfer of weight actions
- The traditional reverence that closes open energy centres in the body to minimize energy depletion and exhaustion

One hypothesis for these similarities relates to the origins of Western classical dance. It is commonly accepted that Western classical ballet was formalized and developed under the governance of King Louis XIV of France, also known as the Sun King. This period in history also represented the height of Franco–Asian exchange. French dignitaries visited Asia, and the French court hosted many visiting Asian sovereigns and their entourages. Louis XIV and the designers of the court of Versailles were impressed and largely influenced by Eastern art and design.

> The idea that the Sun King would be influenced by China and Siam in fashioning his own courtly culture, material environment, and royal image was understandable in the early modern period. . . . These material traces ensured that a distant yet powerful memory of Siam survived in the French imagination into the nineteenth century. (Martin 2015, 662, 666)

If Louis XIV was exposed to Eastern art and the Chinese performing arts, then he would have invariably observed chi kung and kung fu in practice. If we observe the Eastern movement forms from the outside with our Western relationship to art, we would see a series of postures, lines, positions, port de bras and moving sequences; however, we might miss the essential circular nature of the energy flow and the inner processes fundamental to the practice.

APPROPRIATE EFFORT

In our endeavor to achieve the desired line and movement form as seen from the outside, we regularly adopt a more-is-more approach. We strive ceaselessly in Western dance to do *more* – pull up more, turn out more, hold more — with the assumption that more effort, more control, more hours and more repetition will eventually lead to mastery. This more-is-more approach persists even though we have the evidence from sport science that more conscious effort, more conscious control and more physical repetition lead us to more of the same result. It is counterproductive and inefficient and can lead to a global movement dysfunction (Wulf 2007) and pave the way for chronic fatigue, exhaustion and potential injury.

From an Eastern movement perspective, Western dance demands are seen as predominantly *yang*: poised for action, weight forwards on the balls of the feet, muscles engaged and high amounts of muscular control and tension. There is less emphasis in Western dance forms on counterbalancing yin qualities and fewer moments where energy is consciously replenished. An Eastern movement approach teaches that the dual polarities of yin and yang are synergetic and balance one another to facilitate maximum energy flow. Both are equally necessary for the development of stamina and staying power. These polarities are traditionally depicted as contrasts: as a black and white circle, as night and day, or as alkaline and acid. From a movement perspective, we might describe yin movements as expanding, receiving and replenishing; whereas yang movements are high-energy action, contracting muscles and thrusting outward power. Finding the yin moments in dance, in which our system can be replenished and muscular tension released – coming down off demi-pointe and connecting the weight momentarily with the earth, for example – are just as important as the explosive, powerful and sustained yang moments. Without consideration and respect for both, the organism will be rapidly exhausted.

EXPLORATION 3.1 – MOVING THE STONE

Let's take our attention for a moment to our own habitual more-is-more use of effort. Jump up and find a space in your room or simply engage your mind 100 per cent and imagine that right in front of you in the middle of your space is a massive stone – a huge boulder. Without preparation we're going to push the stone as hard as we can for as long as we can and just observe or sense what happens in our body. Are you ready? One . . . two . . . three . . . push . . . push . . . push . . . and? What sort of posture did you adopt? How many muscles did you use? What did that feel like? Were you breathing? Could you have stayed for a long time? Were you effective?

In workshops I ask dancers to reproduce a similar action that requires what they consider maximum power. Spontaneously, without thinking, we move the imaginary stone together as a group, or we split off into pairs and try a traditional arm press contest. Almost all Western dancers spontaneously use a more-is-more approach. They hold their breath completely and adopt a fully contracted, static body posture using maximum muscular engagement and often involving muscle groups essentially irrelevant to the task, such as the face and neck, even the toes. As they run out of steam, energy and oxygen, they collapse and laugh as they realize they were not breathing. They say that it was exhausting, completely unsustainable, not at all effective. Some feel the energy boiling and circling inside their contracted muscles with no place to go. They realize that this more-is-more approach to effort *is* the approach that most of them have learnt in their culture or training and have imprinted in their minds and body as appropriate. It is the 'hologram' of appropriate effort that many Western dancers will adopt when facing challenging dance movements.

EXPLORATION 3.2 – MORE-IS-MORE ARM PRESS

If you would like to do the traditional arm press with another dancer or with your students to clearly identify this learnt imprint of appropriate effort and its associated elements, here are some simple guidelines. One dancer becomes the 'opponent' and the other the active dancer; be sure to swap roles so that each can experience the active role. Ideally both partners should be approximately the same size and corpulence. Both dancers remain in an open, even, bent-leg stance or relaxed demi-plié throughout so that they cannot cheat or push one another by using the weight of the body. The opponent takes the active dancer firmly by the wrist, counts to three and, with maximum effort, tries to fold the dancer's arm towards the dancer's shoulder. The active dancer resists as best they can and simply observes what happens. The objective is not whether the opponent succeeds to fold our arm or not, but simply to observe the process and our body's habitual response.

As the active dancer, were you breathing as you resisted? How many muscles did you engage? What was the quality of the energy? Was the approach effective? Could you have stayed for a long time? Could you have spoken at the same time? Jot down a few key words to describe what you felt, the sensations in the body and the quality of the movement and ask your opponent for any observations about your performance. This will consolidate your awareness so that you can easily recognize this more-is-more pattern of approach when you are dancing. Now swap roles so that your partner becomes the active dancer and can experience the physical outcomes of this approach for themselves.

We frequently see this use of inappropriate effort in Western dance training in a misinformed attempt to produce power, strength and stamina. Using inordinate amounts of muscle engagement in dance for simple tasks such as standing in fifth or balancing in fifth is like dancing with *all the lights on in your house* all of the time – it's extremely uneconomic. We need to wisely select only the *lights* absolutely necessary for the task. Inappropriate muscular engagement drains energy from the system and produces by-products of acids and toxins that in turn need to be removed from the body because they constrict and cramp muscles. A loss of power and stamina is assured when inappropriate effort is used consistently and unnecessary muscle groups are habitually engaged. This alone would change the acidification of the body and lead to solidification of muscles and joints that become more prone to injury.

> . . . any hardness in the body would block the flow of chi (energy) . . . the key to success is having no unnecessary tension in the body. (Brecher 2001, 157).

In chi kung, to bring awareness to unnecessary tension and holding in the body, we might use an analogy such as moving as if we are riding a bicycle. To ride the bicycle efficiently, you need to concentrate your power in the lower body and release unnecessary upper-body tension. You place the hands lightly on the handlebars using only the minimum amount of muscular engagement necessary to steer and to be able to respond to any eventuality the road presents. Similarly, in a simple balance in fifth, I ask dancers to scan their body and *switch off all the lights in the house* that are unnecessary for the task in order to be economic, or I ask them to imagine they have the choice of just three muscles to achieve the balance. So if they are already engaging the face muscles and have tension in the thumbs, that leaves them just one muscle to manage the balance! The number is not important. I am simply drawing their attention to what's appropriate for the task so that they release unnecessary tension and awaken their consciousness to effort.

The less-is-more approach of Eastern movement training uses a series of techniques that lead with the mind and the conscious breath to dissolve blocks and obstacles in the body and mind. These could be muscular hypertension, holding and inappropriate use of effort, or disabling mental dialogue and distraction. Removing these obstacles prepares the path for maximum energy flow, fluidity, speed and precision and permits the development of stamina and power.

FOUNDATIONS OF EASTERN MOVEMENT

Eastern movement is built on three basic foundations that are developed equally to achieve successful, masterful, economic movement. These foundations are (1) alignment and posture, (2) energy and breath and (3) attention and focus (figure 3.1). In Western dance we dedicate many training hours to the first foundation – alignment and posture – to learn how the movement should look from the outside. According to Eastern practice this foundation is just the tip of the iceberg. Two additional foundations require a systematic attention to the inner work of moving and encompass the skills necessary to produce successful movement. So at the same time that alignment and posture are addressed, the synergistic components of coordinated breath, awareness of the flow, quality of energy in movement, intention, attention and focus skills, and a clear mind must also be developed (Jahnke 2002). The three foundations operate in continuous synergy and are to be respected and considered before any movement is executed. The challenge for the dancer then is to develop the capacity to be present and attend to these inner and outer demands simultaneously until they become one experiential movement whole. Let's take a closer look at the concepts involved in this inner work of movement and bring our attention to the second foundation: developing energy and breath.

ENERGY AND BREATH

We can appreciate the importance of the Eastern understanding of the relationship of energy and breath when we realize that in Chinese writing the characters used to represent air, oxygen, breath and inner strength all share the same root symbol representing energy. Breath and energy are understood to come from the same source, suggesting that the mastery of the breath and the quantity of oxygen circulating in our system have a direct impact on the quantity and quality of our energy.

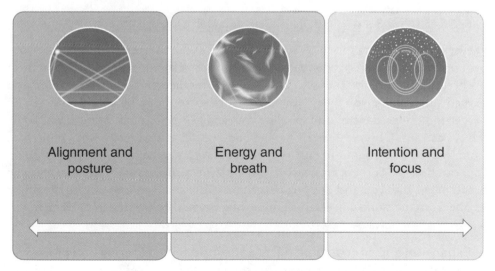

Figure 3.1   Three foundations of an Eastern approach to movement.

Imagine the moment of exchange of oxygen and carbon dioxide happening in each of our billions of cells right now. Each moment of exchange is like a tiny electrical spark. Our body tingles with exchange and bubbles like a golden champagne elixir. The intensity of those billions of sparks literally *is* the intensity of our energy. Some sedentary individuals have a sluggish and slow circulation with poor oxygen potential. Their oxygen flows with few bubbles, like flat champagne, and the rate of exchange is weak and perhaps does not reach all the extremities. The systems of more active people are buzzing with energy exchange as the breath is coordinated and deeply embedded in the rhythm of the movement. Efficient breathing is the key to our vital energy source. Until we bring our attention to the use of the breath, there can be no optimum power or successful renewal of energy in motion.

In traditional Western dance training, the systematic use of the breath is rarely taught. Many of the professional dancers I interviewed shared the same experiences. Their teachers would from time to time say 'breathe'; however, as young dancers they found this instruction vague, especially when it lacked explanation of exactly when, why and how to breathe. When breath *is* introduced in dance, usually relatively late in training, it is typically in relation to performance quality such as the fluidity of port de bras or the practical, big in-breath in preparation for a demanding grand allegro. It is not taught as an integrative tool for mastering technique. As we experienced when moving the stone, the basic challenge for Western dancers is this ill-adapted, more-is-more learnt hologram of maximum effort we have imprinted. In the absence of awareness and alternative training, we hold our breath and we starve our body of oxygen and energy precisely in the most strenuous and demanding moments. This results in suboptimal effectiveness and a loss of power and stamina.

EXPLORATION 3.3 – ATTENTION TO THE BREATH

Whilst you are holding this book and reading, take your attention a moment to your own breathing. Allow tension to drop away from the shoulders and neck and drop the breathing down into the lower body. As you breathe, start to imagine the air and oxygen surrounding you where you sit. You are surrounded by an immense sea of oxygen molecules, dancing and spiraling in an endless continuum, stretching as far as the eye can see. Observe yourself expand and draw in a stream of oxygen molecules from this sea with your in-breath and replace it with a stream of carbon dioxide on your out-breath. If others are nearby, imagine them also expanding in the same way: breathing in with you and drawing oxygen from the same continuum, all breathing as one from the same universal sea of moving oxygen, connected in movement.

Expansion and contraction, filling and emptying, gathering and giving, yin and yang: Eastern practice embraces the simple universal fact that all movement is binary. However complex it might appear, movement is made up of a

---

Attention and Focus in Practice

BREATHING IS EVERYTHING!

Agnès Lopez Rio, professional dancer, teacher, choreographer

Agggh! Breathing, I mean I think no one talks about breathing. In the beginning I think the construction is so difficult, that we all work in apnea! When I remember myself at the beginning, not now, because I had to work on it, I couldn't even see the person in front of me for concentrating so much. My sight was blurry from a lot of tension because if you don't have the strength, you make a lot of extra effort. It's personality as well, but breathing is everything. It's interesting the coordination of the breathing and the movement – but it's weird. You have three types of breathing: chest, lateral and belly. In ballet we like to use the lateral breathing so as not to disturb the verticality, or rather not to have any curves. In the end, this makes you very tense. It's very complicated: Pull this down, close this, don't do that. That's why we are completely rigid and hold our breath. I think when you start to have the verticality of ballet naturally, because you did it all your life, you can start to breathe. My colleagues laugh because I sing the songs of the pianist, but this brings me a sense of normality and a peaceful state of mind. It connects me to my other senses and not only to the perception of effort and working with my body. Singing, breathing naturally and enjoying help me to embrace the effort. And the effort is less.

---

glorious choreography of binary movements. The lungs expand and contract, the heart fills and empties, the muscles release and contract, and there is no other possible movement. Smaller living organisms such as the amoeba or the jellyfish similarly expand and fill their entire bodies and contract as one for propulsion and movement.

THE IN-BREATH

The binary action of the breath is understood and deployed differently in Eastern movement than in many Western movement practices. The in-breath is not considered a powerful moment, but instead a yin action: the refilling and replenishing of potential. We allow breath to flood into the body by expanding cavities. With a yawning-like feeling in the whole body, we make space – opening, expanding and allowing oxygen in with minimum muscular tension.

EXPLORATION 3.4 – THE POTENTIAL OF THE IN-BREATH

Experiment for a moment and fill your body with in-breath using the two different approaches. First take a deep breath in, in preparation as you might have learnt to do by actively drawing breath in through the nose or nose and mouth, and feel how you use your neck and upper-chest muscles. Notice that you perhaps have the feeling of tightening or contraction as you do that, or increased tension in the neck and shoulders or in the diaphragm. Did you also notice that the chest rises, and can you feel the direction of the breath upwards into the head? Retain the in-breath and pause a moment with the breath; notice the feelings in your body. When you can't sustain any longer let go and shake out. Breathing in actively in this way is shallow and ineffective and increases upper-body tension and holding. If used habitually, it can lead to hyperventilation as oxygen remains constricted in the head through upper-body tension. It overstimulates the delicate organs of the brain and nervous system.

Now let's play with the opposite approach: Imagine the chest and the front of the throat released and calm. Imagine that the chest and front of the throat cascade downwards as if someone were stroking down over your face and chest towards your lower body. Start a yawning feeling in the body. Make space, open the throat, expand sideways and downwards, and allow oxygen to flood into the space you created. Imagine the action of the bellows for a fire: As they open, they make space and draw air in. Let's try that again. Begin each time with the calm downwards stroke, and then yawn, expand and make space. I like to imagine the medusa or jellyfish and its amazing ability to effortlessly expand and fill with maximum water potential before propulsion.

THE OUT-BREATH

It is perhaps the name that we give to the out-breath in the West that causes some confusion about its true explosive function. In dance, we often think of the out-breath as the weaker of the two breaths, and we often use it as a moment of release. To call it the out-breath is a misnomer. It's like imagining that the important function of a sports car is the exhaust, which expels waste products whilst ignoring the amazing potential and explosive firing of its engine that occurs in the same action. Of course, just like the sports car, one of the functions of the out-breath is the expulsion of toxins; however, it is also the moment that the motor ignites and explodes into power. As the lungs contract, billions of oxygen molecules surge through the body to the extremities. They spark and exchange in our billions of cells simultaneously, and the potential of the in-breath is transformed into an explosion of yang power.

> Feel how the inhalation gathers . . . potential and how the exhalation diffuses the . . . power of the universe throughout your being. (Jahnke 2002, 44)

Consider the process of coordinating the breath in movement like the process of breathing in singing. An entire singing phrase is one long out-breath. The breath is so fundamental to singers that they study the musical score (the choreography) first and foremost to establish where they need the most power and sustain (out-breath) and where they might replenish their breath (in-breath). Singers search to establish moments of release within the rhythmic demands of the piece to expand and allow oxygen in. Just as in singing, in dance the in-breath and the out-breath cannot function unconsciously, irrespective of the musical, dynamic and power demands of the work. The out-breath can be sustained perhaps four times as long as the in-breath – more depending on the stamina of the artist – without detriment to health. Once a musical or dance piece is prepared in this way, the breath naturally becomes an integral part of the total movement recall.

In Western dance training, when breath *is* mentioned, it typically refers to the conscious use of the in-breath, so we hear 'and take a deep breath in!' As you perhaps experienced in the two approaches to the in-breath in exploration 3.4, actively emphasizing breathing in increases upper-body tension and tightness in the joints and reduces fluidity and readiness for movement. The in-breath is, in fact, a natural reflex action, so whenever we complete a thorough out-breath and then release, the body always automatically takes in oxygen. The out-breath is *not* a reflex action and it, therefore, requires attention to complete a thorough emptying of the lungs. The more we can consciously empty, the more oxygen will naturally refill on the reflex action. The progressive strengthening of the out-breath is an important focus whether training professional dancers for optimum power or working with older adult dancers and those with movement challenges, where supporting a thorough out-breath fosters deeper breathing, lowered heart rate and improved oxygenation, promoting health and well-being.

You can perhaps start to sense the different potential and power of the in- and the out-breath. Let's explore some powerful and sustained movement using the out-breath so that we can experience it directly. Use a slow, sustained out-breath for now, breathing out actively for as long as you can as if you were underwater. You can perform this exploration standing or seated, with the feet flat on the floor and back upright. Prepare a moment by breathing through the spine. Create space between the vertebrae, expanding and contracting the joints themselves with the breathing (Brecher 2001).

EXPLORATION 3.5 – THE POWER OF THE OUT-BREATH

Imagine the yawning sensation and the expansion we created in the second approach to the in-breath when we created space in the body's cavities: in the throat, the lungs, the diaphragm, expanding downwards towards the belly to allow maximum influx. Yawn, expand and allow breath in like a wave to fill all the possible spaces until you

(continued)

EXPLORATION 3.5 *(continued)*

feel full. Suspend with that in-breath a moment . . . three . . . two . . . one . . . turn the wave around. With a slow sustain, send the breath and potential out through all your extremities and beyond, outwards like a star in any direction you want, pressing, reaching, elongating. Keep sending breath out until there's almost no breath left. Can you keep extending? Can you suspend with 'nothing' a moment? And . . . release. Notice the in-breath flood in as a reflex. You didn't have to *do* anything. What did it feel like to continue extending and dancing with no breath? There's so much potential energy and power in the out-breath that we can continue through no-breath and suspend there. We're not holding the breath; there is still outward movement. We're extending with the energy in a kind of dancing apnea (see figure 3.2).

Choose slow, powerful music and experiment with the cycle a few times until it starts to feel fluid . . . pressing, pushing, stretching, spiraling, reaching out into any shape you want through the sustained out-breath. Release and change your position through the transition of the in-breath.

In Eastern practice, the attention is brought to the nature and potential of the breath first through slow movement. The out-breath isn't always slow and sustained of course, and once the application of the breath becomes more automatic, it can be coordinated with the demands of any individual movement or phrase. Coordinating powerful or sustained actions with a conscious out-breath dispels inappropriate effort and tension and maximizes movement efficiency producing fluidity, precision, speed and power. Just as with a piece of music, the choreography might demand the out-breath to be explosive and fast, punching or whipping out into the movement.

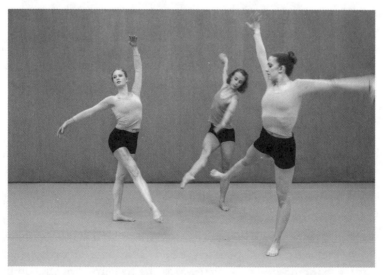

Figure 3.2   Exploring the sustained power of the out-breath. (Emmi, Tehri and Kailey)

Bija Bennett, former professional dancer and international yoga practitioner, suggests to

> Think of your breath as jazz. And you can improvise starting with some fast breaths. Some rapid, soft and punchy breaths. Quick eighth notes of breath. . . . Accenting on the exhale. Finish with some longer, slower, deeper whispering breaths. Lyrical, light, airy-sounding breaths. Then deeper peaceful wave-like breaths. (Bennett 1993)

Although I instruct dancers in the potential use of the breath to enhance their movements, and I give them examples of how to apply them for maximum effect, it's also important to allow time for experimentation and personal choice. I ask them to experiment with the *in* and then the *out* with the same movement and to make their own choice, to find their own power and impetus. The only things that I suggest are *not* options are *not* making a choice or not breathing.

The understanding of breathing in Eastern movement practice goes beyond the binary action of the lungs to include such concepts as a breathing spine, breathing joints, and bone breathing. The breath can in fact be taken to any designated area of the body simply by taking your attention there. This is based on a fundamental of Eastern practice, the understanding that *where the mind will go, blood and energy will follow* (Quian 2017). The focus is on breathing into the area and on expanding the area and dissolving blocks to energy flow (Brecher 2001). The in-breath and the making of space is the yin moment of receiving potential, and the out-breath is the yang moment of propelling energy, oxygen and nutrients through the blocked area and beyond to dissolve holding in muscles and flush out toxins to enhance energy flow. In chapters 4 and 5 we'll explore in more detail potential breath applications to dance-specific challenges.

ATTENTION TO ENERGY

Just as the concepts of oxygen, air, breath and energy in Chinese share the same root symbol, these fundamental elements also share the same universal laws of movement. All fundamental elements, air, energy and including water in all its forms, follow the same universal movement patterns. Moving incessantly, they react in the same flow forms and the same intricate spiraling patterns (Wilkens, Jacobi and Schwenk 2005) (figure 3.3). Whether it concerns the massive movement of the oceans; the air and the weather formations; the steam rising from your coffee cup; a tiny droplet of water from the tap; or indeed the water, air and energy that are dancing through your own human form, all are flowing in these glorious, life-giving spirals. In our whole universe, within and without, there is no such thing as a straight line, a fixed balance, a stable pirouette nor a held moment. All is in perpetual motion, spiraling and

BREATHE LIFE AND ENERGY INTO TECHNIQUE

Raymond Chai, teacher, ballet master, choreographer, former professional dancer

I don't remember ever being taught to breathe or relax. When I was 18 and rehearsing the Bluebird pas de deux and solo, which is a killer, I vaguely remember the teacher saying 'You put the girl down, you walk back and that's your time to breathe'. I finish the pas de deux and I'm walking back, huffing and puffing, when my schoolmate shouts, 'Raymond breathe . . . and breathe . . . and breathe . . .' He kept saying that. And you know, that was probably the first time anyone had said that to me. That has never left me. Just breathe. To get your breath back is to get your energy back.

I didn't like the idea of integrating breath and energy in ballet, though, when I was a dancer. It seemed too esoteric. I was more focused on being technically proficient. If you would have asked me back then to hold, I would have gripped and gone 'grrrrrrr', and I *would* have held the position! Now if students hold, I can clearly see it's static. If there is breathing, the blood has energy and oxygen. If there is relaxation, there is a passage for the energy to flow. Flow, flow, flow . . . when we do that, we *are* controlling and yet at the same time the technique comes alive. I think I always instinctively used energy flow to express and get me through the technical demands; I just never acknowledged as a dancer that the two are so intertwined. If we don't breathe life and energy into technique, dancers become technicians and then it isn't an art. I think this might have come from the Chinese yin and yang, tai chi, martial arts. In my old age I'm going back to my roots without meaning to!

reacting to impetus and intention. To harness this power and its potential, we learn to dance *with* this vast, inevitable, fluid choreography, as if surfing the unpredictable ocean, not by believing, like King Canute, that with enough effort and human determination we might be capable of stopping the waves (Thackeray n.d.).

THE UNIVERSAL ENERGY FIELD

Many ancient Eastern teachings speak of an energy and light continuum that pervades and connects the universe and all the animate beings and inanimate elements within it. These ancient assumptions are consistent with the most recent discoveries of quantum physics and astrophysics scientists (McTaggart 2003). Symbiotic with the continuous sea of oxygen we know to

Figure 3.3   Water-flow forms, after the work of Theodor Schwenk (Wilkens, Jacobi and Schwenk 2005).

be surrounding us is a continuous field of energy made up of electromagnetic energy molecules and known as the electromagnetic or universal energy field. Today, it's no longer a matter of whether we believe in this field of energy or not because it can be perceived by many and photographed and measured by researchers. It's simply a question of learning to understand the nature of the universal energy field and to work *with* rather than against the flow of energy in order to take advantage of this incredible element.

Initial chi kung exercises focus on sensing, touching, gathering, condensing, stretching, releasing, playing and dancing through this external energy field until we start to become aware of its movement and to respect its qualities and its speed. Learning to perceive the flow of energy around and through our movements and beyond is one of the potential sensory external attentional focus types we identified on the spectrum of EF possibilities (figure 2.3). When learning these foundational skills, we often use other analogies for the energy field: metaphorical imagery such as moving through a large body of water because water shares the same universal movement patterns as energy. We imagine the water reacting to our own movements and swirling around our body, or we imagine the insistent air bubbles of massage jets in a warm thermal bath as they bombard our skin surface or we gather millions of dancing champagne-like energy bubbles and try to contain their movements within our arms. Energy, by its very nature, is never still.

EXPLORATION 3.6 – ATTENTION TO THE UNIVERSAL ENERGY FIELD

Let's experiment and begin to play with the universal energy field. As you move, aim always to have just a little air circulating around the body, under the arms, between the fingers, even when you are at rest. This maximizes the surface in contact with the universal energy field and affects the amount of energy that can flow through you. If we close the fingers tight, press our arms down to our sides or touch our own body in any way, we short-circuit and reduce potential energy flow. Choose your favourite relaxing music to accompany you. Take an open parallel position, sink into the 'water' and let your breathing become calm and natural like a wave:

3.6(a) – Gathering Energy

Sensitize the hands a moment by rubbing the palms together quickly, making friction as if you were cold. Now throw them wide out to the side and float the arms on the surface of the 'water', without muscular effort. Imagine all the millions of energy molecules in this universal field, dancing like golden champagne bubbles. We're going to gather an armful of dancing energy molecules. Breathing naturally, draw the palms very slowly towards each other as if you want to scoop up as many as possible to make a kind of energy snowball. Palm facing palm, fingers facing fingers, draw them slowly together. At a certain point, you might start to notice a tingling sensation between your palms. It doesn't matter if this is at beach ball size or tennis ball size. Imagine the millions of energy molecules that are condensed between your palms still dancing away. As a test, give them a gentle press inwards and you perhaps will notice your hands bounce open a little from the pressure of the dancing molecules.

Release any tension and see if you can move for a moment with that dancing ball of energy and maintain that tingling sensation between your palms. When do you lose the tingling sensation? What did you do? Can you recover the sensations? After a count of three, recycle all those dancing molecules in the ground. One . . . two . . . three . . . and throw them off into the earth with a large out-breath. Thank them for playing with you, and shake them off your fingers because energy is a little sticky. You're ready to throw your arms wide again.

3.6(b) – Stretching Energy

Moving on, let's explore some of the qualities of energy. Gather energy as you did before by drawing your arms and hands towards each other until you have a condensed ball of dancing molecules. Begin to move and play. Allow your body to be fluid as it follows the movement of the energy without tension. Now slowly, begin to stretch the energy in any direction you want. Imagine the sticky energy stretching between the palms of your hands like sticky honey as you draw your hands away from one another. If you draw one hand towards the sky and one towards the earth, how far can you go and still feel or imagine the threads of honey between your hands before they dissolve? Breathe out and firmly squash or condense the energy molecules back together into the ball between your hands and move freely with the condensed ball of moving energy. When you recover the tingling sensations, take a slow stretch in another direction and focus on the tingling sensations between your palms and the threads of honey-like energy. When you are ready, recycle all those dancing molecules in the ground as you did before. One . . . two . . . three . . . and throw the breath out and shake the molecules off into the earth.

Before you move on, notice the sensations in your body. What are you feeling? Do you feel lighter? Brighter? Are you smiling? Do you feel tingling and heat in the hands? Over the upper body? Down through the legs? These sensations are increased circulation, oxygen and energy flow within and around the body. *Where the mind will go, energy, blood, circulation and oxygen will follow* (Quian 2017).

Eventually, let the two parts of the exploration flow one into another so that you have a continuous moment of play and improvisation with the universal energy field. The pace is slow at first, giving you time to perceive and observe the sensations. Revisiting this energy play regularly will increase your sensitivity to energy flow and consolidate your proprioceptive sensations. As you become more fluent, you will find that you can move faster and more dynamically and still sense the moving energy and the honey-like threads between your movements. You might integrate this moment of play immediately into morning pliés and port de bras.

In the West, we often just use one generic term for *energy* as we might use the term *water*. However with *water* we understand that it has many forms, qualities and sources: the water of the ocean, the rain, a gushing river, a trickling stream, a spring, a stagnant pond, rising steam. Likewise, in Eastern terms there are many forms, qualities and sources of *energy*, the animating life force known as chi. Energy may be drawn from the universal energy field, it may be of our human energy field, such as the daily acquired-chi generated directly from the food we eat, or it might be inherited-chi from our family and our birth, our original essential energy (Dirlam Ching and Ching 2007).

THE HUMAN ENERGY FIELD

What is commonly referred to as the *human energy field* is not in fact separate or a different energy from that of the universal energy field. The term simply refers to the field of energy directly surrounding an individual. The human energy field is coloured by all the aspects specific to that individual and their biography. Their history and accumulated lived experiences, physical health, psychological and emotional state, and hereditary energy all inform the nature and quality of an individual's human energy field. Some sensitive individuals can see and read the information we carry with us in the human energy field, as if it were our own detailed hard disk. It is often described as a body of light that surrounds and interpenetrates the physical body and commonly referred to as the 'aura' (Brennen 1988). This human energy or electromagnetic field can also be photographed using a technique known as Kirlian photography that shows different colour spectrum tendencies and patterns according to the individual and their immediate emotions and state of mind.

Energy knows no boundaries and dances through and around us. Despite our own sense of solidity and permanence, we are in fact not solid at all. 'You *are* an electric field – a giant electric field that holds your atoms together and that uses other electric fields to talk to other bits of yourself . . . it is the only way you can possibly exist as a coherent entity!' explains Dr Jack Fraser, astrophysics tutor at Oxford University (Fraser 2017). We are a constantly changing choreography of dancing atoms.

According to science reporter Ali Sundermier, we are made up of 99.9 per cent space – the same limitless space we encounter in outer space. 'Since the meat of your atoms is nestled away in nuclei, when you "touch" someone (or something), you aren't actually feeling their atoms. What you're feeling is the electromagnetic force of your electrons pushing away their electrons' (Sundermier 2016, para. 19). The idea that we are permeable, fluid beings made up of inner space, animated by dancing electricity is an inspirational and liberating image I find for transforming my own dance practice.

A common Western thought is that our energy is somehow personal to us or is limited to the energy drawn from the food we eat. Many people imagine that when we make an effort and produce force, we are depleting our own personal energy reserves and that once exhausted, they are empty. One of the sources of our daily energy is, of course, the nutrients from the food we take in; however, it's far from the only source. It's important to know how to replenish the energy we take from the universal energy field, for example, and to keep it circulating. Energy is not personal and is not exhausted if we learn to consciously renew and replenish the energy in our organism whilst in motion.

The study of chi kung then is simply the study of energy and how to move and dance with it for optimum efficiency. Chi kung promotes the free flow of energy throughout the body and the organs and ensures that it can powerfully course like water through a clear conduit. The clearer the conduit, free of tension and toxins, the greater the potential volume of energy that can flow through the body. Wherever energy is not flowing optimally – because of holding or unnecessary muscular or mental tension – will be a potential area of weakness. If tension is left unaddressed to become chronic, the resulting energy block, exacerbated by the lack of adequate circulation and oxygenation, will produce discomfort and will ultimately be prone to disease. As soon as we release holding and make space, fresh energy rushes in like sea water at the beach as we build our sandcastle. See chapter 5 and exploration 5.2 for more about replenishing energy from the universal energy field.

ENERGY IN MOTION

Energy and its movement are easiest to sense initially in the upper body and in the hands, arms and fingers, so the energy work of chi kung commences with a series of basic port de bras. As with the gathering and stretching energy exploration we did earlier (exploration 3.6), these ports de bras gather energy in the lower body and then lift it and lower it throughout the body, using the coordinated breath to literally pump the energy through the organs, the muscles and beyond. The ports de bras focus around three principal energy centres in the body: lower, middle and upper. A lower-body energy centre, or dan tien, corresponds approximately to the area defined by bras bas in classical ballet. Energy for action is continually replenished and stored in this lower energy centre (Brecher 2001). All exercises begin and end with gathering and lowering energy into this part of the body where energy may be safely stored. A middle energy centre corresponds approximately to the area defined by first position in classical ballet, surrounding the solar plexus and heart area. An upper energy centre is located in the brain area and is associated with the elevated consciousness and spirit that connects to the universe through the top of the head, or crown (Rodell 2017). This upper energy centre corresponds to the area encircled by the arms in classical fifth position, or couronne.

Similar to a classical ballet port de bras, the chi kung exercises commence with a preparatory 'breathing arm' that provides a quiet, neutral moment allowing the dancer to consciously gather energy, to still the mind and bring their attention into the present moment and to the task at hand. The series of chi kung ports de bras progressively gather and lift energy from the lower energy centre (bras bas) first to the middle energy center – the solar plexus and heart centre (first position), which is associated with the emotions. The lifted energy activates the area and then the port de bras opens to give this heart energy back into the energy field (a classical demi-port de bras). Later the port de bras takes the energy higher through the body, past the delicate organs of the nervous system, the eyes and the brain to the crown energy centre and activates this higher energy (fifth position, or couronne). Lifted energy is released towards heaven back into the universe and then the arms slowly lower through a position of resting on the water of a stream (second position) to gather fresh energy and draw it safely back in the lower energy centre, dan tien (bras bas, a classical full port de bras). Chapter 4 (exploration 4.1) revisits the origins of the classical port de bras and its relationship to energy and breath in more detail.

The energy we gather in a port de bras not only circles and dances within the space encircled by the arms but also passes effortlessly through the 99.9 per cent space that is our body. It activates adjacent body areas, charging the energy centre, to circle around and down through the arms themselves, jumping the void between the fingertips, and connecting and completing the circle (figure 3.4). As we experienced in exploration 3.6b, energy has a sticky quality, and honey-like threads can be experienced as we draw the arms away from one another in any position (e.g., as we move slowly from a classical first to second position of the arms or from fifth to fourth position). All ports de bras connect moving energy clearly between the lower, heart and crown energy centres and propel it through the extension of the limbs and beyond.

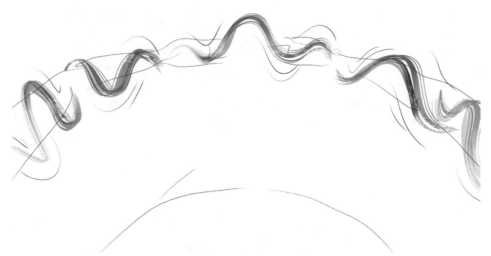

Figure 3.4   Circling energy jumps the void, connecting and completing the circle.

Once we become sensitive to the flow of energy in port de bras, movement progression is used to increase the energy flow and pressure through the body. For example, movement sequences use a progressively deeper lowering of the body (demi-plié or full plié) because the lowering increases the pressure of the energy flow and circulation. The deeper the plié, the greater the counterenergy pressure rising through the body (Kam Chuen 1991).

Later, in more advanced movement sequences, chi kung movement shifts the weight forwards from a whole-foot, even stance that is used to promote the health and balance of our organism onto the ball of the foot, or demi-pointe. This progression further increases energy pressure and develops explosive power. Chi kung Master Lam Kam Chuen explains that the feet have a remarkable structure that can bear weight and yet at the same time remain sensitive and spring-like, reacting to pressure like those of a cat. When pressure is applied downwards into the earth, a chain reaction occurs, like a spring that carries on upwards and affects the whole structure of the body. This action develops and pumps explosive energy through the system (Kam Chuen 2003). Movement sequences continue to coordinate the action of the breath: the in-breath replenishing potential and the out-breath activating and pumping energy through the body and beyond. Once this breathing coordination becomes more fluent, movement progresses to another level to direct energy flow simply with the mind rather than relying on the breath pattern as an energy pump. Eventually we aim to move energy with our clear intention, attention and focus on the desired effect of the movement (EF). The foundations of breath and energy and of attention and focus are inseparable in Eastern movement practice. Each element is as essential as another, working synergistically to facilitate powerful, effective and efficient movement.

ATTENTION AND FOCUS

The recent body of attentional focus research concurs with Eastern movement practice to suggest that the ability to clear the mind and focus the attention far from self-related concerns enhances balance, fluidity, speed, precision, power, stamina, perception, multitasking and artistry (Mornell and Wulf 2019). Eastern teaching associates these performance benefits with the focus of movement initiation itself. Movement may be initiated in two ways: it may be mind-led, with the attention focused on the effect, the quality or the desired outcome of the movement (as in EF), or it may be muscle-led, with attention on the conscious control of the body and a focus on body part or muscle-led initiation (as in IF). Both initiations are movement control strategies; however, according to chi kung practice, mind-led (EF) has significant advantages over muscle-led (IF).

To appreciate both approaches, imagine a cat watching an annoying house fly buzzing about his head and ears. He's very still, following the movement of the fly. Suddenly, without warning, he lashes out. With a lighting quick, fluid, economic, precise and effective movement, he gets the fly. The cat is using a mind-led external focus on the effect of his movement. His focus and intention is simply to get the fly. Now imagine that the cat could think and analyse his movement and consciously instruct his own body. If he could tell himself to prepare, engage his core muscles, raise his foreleg, open his claws and swipe with the paw, his movement would be slow and inconsistent and he would use way too much muscular engagement. He would miss the fly every time. However absurd the image of the thinking cat might be, this *is* the initiation and control approach that many dancers adopt during challenging dance movement.

These two distinct movement initiations promote two very different qualities of energy that are clearly defined in the martial arts. When we allow the mind to lead, we promote what is known as *jin energy*. Jin movements require no muscular preparation and respond to the mind's attention with a lightning quick, reflexive action. There is seemingly no delay in the signal from brain to body, and energy flows efficiently out through the relaxed movement. A jin movement is efficient as it uses the minimum muscular engagement necessary for maximum force production appropriate to the task. This mind-led jin approach corresponds to the description of an external attentional focus in human movement science terminology, sharing the same evidenced benefits: It is fast, economic, consistent, precise and powerful and facilitates stamina and staying power. To move with jin energy, we pay attention to our sensations and *listen with the skin* according to Master Dennis Watts, president of the Tai Chi Association of Australia. 'We need to be aware that mind is leading the Chi (energy) . . . and not to push our form, for to do so will cause the body to be scattered and the movements uncoordinated' (Watts n.d., para. 5).

Movement initiated and led from the body parts or muscles, provoking what is termed *li energy*, has a delay whilst the body and brain communicate – a moment of preparation and a drawing back for muscular engagement. Someone who habitually uses li energy can become visibly muscular or muscle bound according to Eastern practice as they focus their attention on the muscles. Li energy corresponds to the evidenced effects of an internal attentional focus as defined in human movement science: It is slower to react and produces inconsistent movements that waste energy and are easily exhausted, resulting in tired, sore muscles. According to Eastern teachings there *are* occasions when it might be necessary to initiate movement from the muscles; however, this should be done as a conscious choice, with caution because it is always energetically draining and depleting for the body.

> First we must loosen the body and then expand across each joint. If you listen to the movement and then coordinate your breath, plus visualize the application of the movement, you should feel the body slightly expand in all directions. . . . (Watts n.d., para 8)

Even if we try consciously to instruct our muscles to relax, we can create more tension in the body. Breath, space and energy cannot be forced. We cannot control them by making *more* effort; we must simply *allow* space and *allow* energy to flow as we dance. Say the word *allow* to yourself and notice what happens in your body. As we allow space, we gently release and expand in all directions without effort. Fresh energy will naturally flow into this space and follow the path of least resistance (Brecher 2001).

Wayne McGregor, resident choreographer of The Royal Ballet, observes that

> . . . one of the beautiful things about those practices where attention actually reconnects you with your own body . . . where you do a body scan . . . and it makes you literally taller. It's not imagining you are taller. It actually creates space in your vertebrae and your hips and your legs and your joints and at the end of it you feel that the volume of your body inhabits the space in a very different way. (Watson 2017, 244)

ALLOWING THE MIND TO LEAD

Let's revisit exploration 3.2, the more-is-more arm press that we did earlier, and this time let's do it differently. We will take the same exercise but this time with a less-is-more approach, allowing the mind to lead and guide the attention in order to clearly identify the appropriate effort of this approach and the associated response of the body.

EXPLORATION 3.7 – LESS-IS-MORE ARM PRESS

In this exploration one dancer becomes the 'opponent' and the other the active dancer as before. Be sure to swap roles so that each can experience the sensations of the active role. Ideally both partners should be approximately the same size and corpulence. Both dancers take an open, active stance as before and sink down into an easy demi-plié. Aim to remain in an even demi-plié throughout so that neither one can cheat or push with the weight of the body. The opponent takes the active dancer firmly by the wrist and counts to three as before and uses their maximum more-is-more effort to try to fold the arm towards the active dancer's shoulder.

As the active dancer you need to prepare the attention and focus for this mind-led movement. Imagine that your arm has a fish-like quality – that is to say, imagine that it is energized, powerful and yet 'swimming' or fluid with breathing joints and is responsive to the external movement of energy or 'water'. You might imagine a powerful salmon that is determined, focused and yet able to respond to its external element with lightning speed.

Open the fist and direct energy out continuously through the arm, the breathing joints and the fingers (figure 3.5). Let them be free of tension so that maximum energy can flow. Direct the fluid energy as far away as you can imagine. Look for a clear path for this energy and aim out to the trees or to the far wall, rather than straight through your partner or other dancers. Ask your opponent to check that your arm is fluid, that your shoulders, biceps and triceps are not tense or contracted and that your elbow and wrist are breathing and fluid. Take a few natural breaths low in the body to gather energy. Keep your attention 100 per cent on the direction of the outward flowing energy and its trajectory to the tree or the wall and beyond. Trust the experience. Are you ready?

Three . . . two . . . one . . . go. Breathe easy and naturally. Maintain your clear focus. No need to *do* anything else. Breathe. Filter out your partner's more-is-more efforts and breathlessness. Focus on sending fluid energy out with a fish-like quality. Allow the joints to breathe. Nothing else – only energy flowing outward . . . and . . . sustain . . . and release.

How did you get on? What did you observe in your body? Were you breathing? How many

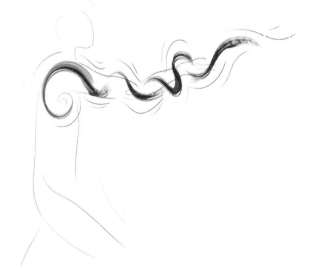

Figure 3.5   Mind-led, less-is-more arm press.

(continued)

muscles were you using this time? How did this compare to the more-is-more arm press (exploration 3.2)? Was it an effort? Could you have sustained it for a long time? Could you have spoken? Ask your opponent to share what they observed, the quality of the movement and the energy they sensed. Was it shaky or constant? How was your power this time?

Jot down a few key words to describe the experience to consolidate the associated sensations and proprioceptive sense of effort in this less-is-more approach so that you can easily recall all aspects of this mind-led approach when dancing. Now swap roles and sense again as the opponent this time. Both the active and the opponent role are rich in implicit learning opportunities to consolidate our awareness of appropriate effort.

In attention and focus workshops I usually explore muscle-led more-is-more arm press (exploration 3.2) and then immediately mind-led less-is-more arm press (exploration 3.7) so that dancers can feel and compare the quality of the effort and the effectiveness of the two approaches: the more-is-more approach of leading with the muscles and the less-is-more approach of allowing the mind to lead. A stunned silence typically hits the room as many dancers experience for the first time a powerful, constant, stable movement achieved without effort. In the silence, the potential of this discovery dawns on the dancers and they begin to anticipate how they will apply a less-is-more approach to dance practice.

The mind-led, less-is-more image of a fish-like quality can be effectively applied to any movement to promote the use of minimum effort and maximum energy flow and power. So we might aim for fish-like arms, or legs or spine. Eastern movement practice frequently uses metaphorical images of animals such as a bird, a tiger, a cat or a fish to guide the mind and promote the desired movement qualities embodied by the image, providing a perfect external focus of attention.

Initially, mind-led energy flow is developed through the upper body, arms and hands because this area tends to be more sensitive and responsive. Applying this same approach to the more muscular lower body and legs may take a little practice, as when learning any new language. We need first to attend to releasing tension and allowing space in the powerful joints of the hips and lower back in order to be able to sense the energy flow; however, some immediate benefits such as a sense of lightness, economy and ease of movement and improved stability and increased range of motion can be experienced. In chapter 4 you'll find dance-specific explorations of a less-is-more approach to posture and balance, and the fish-like quality of the spine and the unfolding leg – developpé.

One simple and yet effective idea we might adopt from an Eastern approach that will assist with this lower-body sensitization is the different understanding of the role of each leg in movement. The guiding principle in any Eastern movement is the respect for the standing leg and the standing side no matter what the demands of the movement are. The standing leg then is considered the *working* leg and it is referred to as the *full leg*. It is full of the responsibility to support the movement, and it's full of energy, pressure, blood flow and connection to the earth. Without this respect and connection, any movement is compromised. The free leg in the air is considered the *playing* leg and is referred to as the *empty leg* because it is not weight bearing and is free to play and respond. This simple reversal of terminology, *working and playing leg* or *full and empty leg,* shifts our habitual focus away from the non-weight-bearing leg in the air back onto our essential support. Adopting this terminology and shifting the focus of attention in this way has an immediate impact not only on stability and balance but also on the lightness and the efficiency of the actions of both legs.

If movement should be mind-led, then that means that what goes on in our mind and with our attention is of utmost importance because it has a direct impact on our physical performance. It means that there is no such thing as an idle thought. If, *where the mind will go, blood and energy follow* (Quian 2017), then all of those millisecond thoughts that we have that flash past and all that self-talk that occurs that is irrelevant to the task are simply distracting and undermining our optimal performance.

In Eastern movement practice, the use of the mind and the process of attention are trained and developed as an integral part of movement learning. Managing those darting thoughts and self-talk is referred to as the *no-mind principle*. This does not refer to trying to achieve a mindless state – quite the reverse. In the no-mind state, we filter the mind of extraneous information and distracting thoughts, whether negative or positive, and create space. The spacious mind is charged with energy and is attentive and receptive in the present moment. Like the concept of the 'empty' limb, we make space in the mind so that maximum energy can flow. Because we are all human, we all have days or performances where we don't seem able to keep the self-talk and information overload clear from our mind. This is not a process that we can control with *more* effort. We start by becoming aware of our wandering attention and of irrelevant or critical thoughts and then we can choose to reset the mind and bring our attention back to the present moment, back to the movement effect, the breath and the sensations (Taylor 2015). The more we practise this awareness, the more agile our ability to reset and bring our mind to a quiet, focused attention.

So start by simply becoming aware of the movement of your own attention and focus whilst you are dancing and notice when thoughts habitually interrupt. Awareness is already 50 per cent of the journey towards heightening these skills. When you are dancing, do your thoughts tend to go back to a past event? For example, do you criticize yourself for something you have just done or not done in that exercise? Or do you habitually take your mind to the future and worry about whether you will be able to manage something that's yet to come? Perhaps you do both. How easy is it for you to stay with your chosen attentional focus, image or proprioceptive sensation to support your present movement without thoughts interrupting? For a movement to be successful, we aim to be 100 per cent in the present moment with the mind and body full with maximum energy. Additional self-talk that takes the attention backwards to the past or forwards to the future drains vital energy from the present moment and, therefore, undermines results. *Where the mind will go, blood and energy will follow* (Quian 2017). We reduce our power, both physical and mental, when our mind is not attending to *this* moment, and we diminish our sensory capacity to perceive and react.

The mind is our most powerful resource, and it is essential as a dancer – just as it is in sports – that we train our ability to attend to its processes and harness its full potential. In chapter 5 you'll find explorations and ideas to support and strengthen your attentional skills.

DISTANCE EFFECT

In Eastern movement practice, physical and mental performance is enhanced progressively by the use of a distant attention and focus that brings additional benefits to performance as identified in the distance effect of human movement science research (chapter 2). The mind and the attention are shifted onto increasingly distant foci and objectives. For example, initial focus may be on the pressure we feel when pushing the floor to rise, and this can be gradually progressed to imagine the pressure and energy continuing further down into the earth. Or when making space in the spine, we can imagine sending energy through the crown to the ceiling and then progressively extend energy towards the sky. The further away we project the effect of the movement, the greater the flow of energy through our movement, as if the energy tries to follow our mind to reach our distant point of attention. All the benefits of a focus on the effect of the movement (EF) – balance, precision, fluidity, power, stamina, perception and artistry – are incrementally enhanced the further away we project our attention from the self (figure 3.6). One technique circulates the energy from the lower body in progressively widening orbits around the human energy field and beyond to orbit as far out as the solar system to expand the energy flow (Kam Chuen 1991). The orbiting energy then reverses its direction and is drawn back towards the human energy field, condensing energy back into the lower energy centre of the body.

EXPLORATION 3.8 – DISTANT ATTENTION – ENHANCING ENERGY

To develop the use of distant attention, you can progress exploration 3.6*b* by drawing your hands further away from each other in the stretch until the energy threads completely dissolve. Press up towards the sky with one hand and downwards to the earth with the other. Breathe out and connect a moment between earth and sky, and pause a moment extending out in both directions (figure 3.6). As you release, immediately condense thousands of energy molecules together into your energy ball and lower-body energy centre to increase the energy flow through your body.

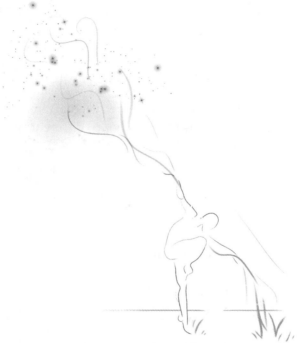

Figure 3.6   Distant attention – connecting earth and sky.

Some advanced forms of Eastern martial arts use these attentional techniques to expand and contract the energy field around the body in the same way, condensing the surrounding energy molecules in the human energy field for use in combat.

As we begin to incorporate these foundational attention and energy concepts into dance practice in the next chapter, perhaps start with the attention closer to the human energy field by using the real, tangible and sensory EF: Attend to the pressure of the floor, to a proprioceptive sensation, to the threads connecting energy between the limbs, for example. Once you become more fluent at directing your attention onto the effect or the outcome of the movement, gradually introduce the element of distance using metaphorical imagery as a progression to enjoy the increased physical and mental benefits. Aim for the stars in your dance practice and allow the mind to assure the energy and the power for you to reach them.

We are sculptors of air, energy, breath and light — encircling and dancing through us and beyond.

We envelop and sculpt energy in the moment, in every present moment with our intention, attention and focus.

Dance is not of the body. It is not the physical movements nor the shapes that can be observed or captured. This is to miss the vital essence of what we do. To capture what appears solid and tangible is to miss the flow of mind, energy, electricity, connection, artistry.

Choreographer Wayne McGregor reflects that

There's lots of ways that you can mediate between attention and intention and you have to understand that they are different and then you can play them like an instrument. (Watson 2017, 243)

REFLECTION PROMPTS

We covered a lot of new concepts and ideas in a short introductory chapter! Before we move on to explore how these translate to support your dance training and performance, take a moment to review the observations you jotted down after each exploration in the chapter. I'm sure some intuitive, creative ideas popped up as well whilst you were reading – be sure to note those down too for use in your dancing.

Here are some reflective questions to prompt your thoughts:

- What did you learn that was totally new?
- Did any aspect of your understanding change whilst reading this chapter?
- Did you have any aha! moments that revealed to you how these concepts might translate to your dance practice or how you might apply these ideas? Are there any you can integrate immediately into class or teaching?

The Eastern study of the role of the breath and energy and attention and focus is a vast, rich body of knowledge and ancient wisdom. I have been able to touch only the surface here and make the most basic introduction to the concepts that I consider most relevant to dance practice. If these concepts have sparked an interest, then explore and follow up using some of the sources listed in the references to read more about the subject. Deepening your understanding of energy, breath, attention and focus will have an immediate and lasting effect on your dance practice and enrich your unique artistry.

CHAPTER

4

ATTENTIONAL FOCUS: ENHANCING POWER, PRECISION AND ARTISTRY

. . . perceive the extraordinary in the ordinary by changing not the world, but the eyes that look.

Jane Hirschfield (quoted in Watson 2017, 142)

*A*rtists of multiple disciplines describe their process as one of bringing their attention consistently to the everyday, the familiar, the mundane. This discipline requires a constant revisiting, a daily process of defamiliarization that has the power to reach through habitual ways of seeing and doing, reach beyond the known to look and experience the familiar with fresh eyes.

In the art of dance, we too revisit the body, our instrument, every morning. Reduced to its most basic, our instrument comprises two arms, two legs, a torso and a head. We reinvent the infinite combinations over and over in our lifelong journey of exploration and performing. Imagine that as an artist we have perhaps started our day with more than 10,000 morning pliés. We may believe that we now *know* our technique and our body. Our daily practice has become familiar and perhaps habitual. Habit and familiarization – believing we already know or approaching the movement the way we always have done – means that we cease to draw our attention to the movement in *this* moment. This overfamiliarization is an obstacle to progress in our art, to moving beyond our plateau to reach our optimal dancing best. Attend to the process of daily **defamiliarization**.

When we can be 100 per cent in the moment or present in the studio – paying attention to our experiences, to our sensations, to the external world and reexploring the possibilities of our instrument every day – then new, hitherto unimagined possibilities and potential unfold. It's the ability to revisit and attend to the activity afresh – to experience that 10,000th plié as if for the very first time, to give space to and guide the attention – that renews energy and power, ensuring speed, precision and fluidity and enabling artistry.

In this chapter we revisit some of the fundamentals of our daily practice and approach them with fresh eyes by integrating a few of the ancient and recent scientific attention and focus ideas we have explored so far. We'll experience their potential application to foundations such as posture, port de bras, turnout and balance and then to the specific challenges of dance skills such as the fluid sustain of adage; the dynamic balance of turns and pirouettes; and the precision, speed and explosive power of jumps and allegro. Each example is simply a taster to spark your own creativity. The possibilities for shifting your attention away from conscious, self-related, body control to an external focus of attention, of choosing to attend to the mind, the imagery, the quality of energy and the cohesive integration of the breath, are infinite.

Sorella Englund, international ballet master and coach at The Royal Danish Ballet, describes exactly the need for such attention and *presence* when performing *La Sylphide*:

> . . . you have to learn to *be* more and *do* less. That's the hard thing, because as a dancer you always think it's very boring if you're not *doing* a lot. But you have to have the guts to do less and be incredibly present. (Flatow n.d., para. 5)

Be more and *do* less: This is the essence of an Eastern movement approach or an external focus of attention (EF) approach and contrasts with an internal focus of attention (IF) approach. Prioritizing *doing* (IF) rather than *being* (EF) comes at the expense of efficient movement as we shut down in-the-moment perceptive skills that deliver body wisdom and autonomous solutions to our dancing challenges. So, suspend your disbelief, welcome the new challenge of defamiliarization with curiosity and enjoy the process and the results!

REVISITING THE FOUNDATIONS OF DANCE

Before we embark on the process of defamiliarization from our habitual approach to the foundations of dance, let's recap briefly what we covered in chapters 2 and 3 and how we might potentially guide our attention and our focus. It's not possible to attend to all these new potential foci at once; this would simply add to your dancing to-do list and exacerbate your information overload. Imagine these complementary attentional ideas rather as your palette of alternative *colours*: your tools to choose from that will enable you to revisit the known and be 100 per cent present in your dancing. They will support and lighten the physical demands of the technique and boost your capacity to learn, and at the same time will free up your cognitive reserve for interpretation and artistry.

Here are a few of the attentional focus tools we have looked at so far:

- Choose an EF control strategy and guide your attention systematically onto the desired movement effect, objective or quality using any of the EF possibilities (in figure 2.3) to provide fast jin energy and optimal, reflexive movement organization. As we saw in chapter 3, *mind first – muscles follow*.

- Be 100 per cent present in the moment and in the movement with the EF, whether you're using a real, physical object as a focus, a tangible element or sensory feedback and imaginary foci.

- Make space and *allow* movement. Seek constantly to identify and dissolve unnecessary holding or tension in the body or inappropriate effort in a movement to allow optimal energy flow throughout.

- Dance with the minimal muscular engagement possible for maximal coherence, speed, fluidity and stamina.

- Attend to the easy flow of the breath by expanding, making space and allowing potential in and maximizing the explosive power or the sustain of the 'out'.

- Dance with the flow of the breath and coordinate, like music, with the demands of the movement for optimum effect.

- Draw energy from the universal energy field, ensuring a constant source to the nervous system and the organs, lifting and enlivening the joints.
- Guide, play, sculp and dance with the energy through the movements and beyond for optimum power and responsive artistry.

Choreographer William Forsythe reflects on physical thinking whilst in the studio at The National Ballet of Canada. 'Dancers are very intentional by the nature of the practice', he observes. However, the important question that he poses dancers is, 'how do you direct attention to your intention?' (National Ballet of Canada 2019).

POSTURE

In a typical dance posture, we look for a lifted, lengthened spine, a neutral or balanced pelvis and a lengthened occipital bone. If we use muscular force to achieve the length and lift of the basic posture, then the posture becomes tense and rigid before we even begin to move. This is far from the ideal starting place for fluid, energized action. In Eastern movement practice, basic posture also has the same requirements that seek a straightened and elongated spine, a lengthened sacrum and occipital bone area. In Eastern movement, this is desired because the spine is known to be the body's 'energy highway' that transports energy from the lower-body energy centre where it is stored to serve the vital organs and the nervous system. Maximum 'breathing' space is sought between the joints of the vertebrae to permit optimum energy flow and space for the organs to function. We seek a fish-like, strong yet fluid spine, breathing and coursing with energy and ready for any movement eventuality. Eastern practice uses jin energy, led by the mind and attention, to achieve this effortless support without tension. Jin energy has the characteristic of providing resistance like a spring. It is described as supportive and balanced and yet promotes the minimum effort in movement response. As substantial energy is gathered in the lower body (dan tien or bras bas), tai chi Master Dennis Watts explains, there is a corresponding rise of upward energy from the inside to the crown and beyond like a spring, which keeps the body centred and aligned (Watts n.d.). The upper body and head are led upwards by this rising energy and this creates the sensation of being suspended from the crown, the first yang pressure point in traditional Eastern medicine. This idea of being suspended from the crown is an image that we use frequently in dance.

An exercise called *the large circulation of energy* uses the mind to lead energy in a two-directional, figure-8 action from the earth upwards and from the universe downwards. This produces the two-way directional pull that we also refer to in dance. It promotes an ideal posture without muscular tension. See figure 4.1. With an in-breath, energy is drawn up from the earth through the front of the legs, passed through the lower-body energy centre and guided forcefully up the back, lifting the spine and occipital area to flow out through the crown and beyond into the universe. With an out-breath, energy is drawn down across the front of the body to cascade across the face and chest, pass again through the lower energy centre and descend, promoting a feeling of drawing down the back of the legs into the earth. This figure-8 movement of universal energy lengthens and corrects posture in one global externally focused idea, energizing the body and producing this sensation of a gentle, yet consistent, two-way postural pull. This large circulation of energy can be practiced at any point using just the mind to lead the energy, independent of the pumping action of the breath. Another variation, the small circulation of energy, leads energy with the mind to circle around the body. The energy is led up through the spine and occipital bone, around the crown, then to flow down, softening the front of the body and then on around, powerfully up through the spine again. (See exploration 5.3.) This smaller circulation can also be done at any time during movement to ensure this fluid, effortless lift and renewal of energy throughout our dancing. (See exploration 5.4 for more postural foci.)

TURNOUT – ROTATION

The original objective of the outward rotation of the legs used extensively in dance was to allow freedom of movement, provide greater stability in motion and enhance the explosive potential of preparatory movements. The outward rotation of the legs is not simply an aesthetic peculiarity of classical ballet, but it's a practical adaptation of the human stance seen in many other movement forms such as the Eastern martial arts and the traditional sport of fencing. If we imagine this outward rotation, or turnout, as a position

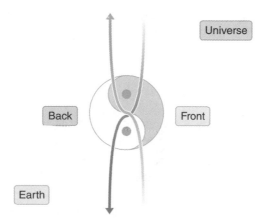

Figure 4.1   The large circulation of energy for effortless two-way postural support.

of the lower limbs with a fixed end point, then, as we experienced with the posture, we will engage inappropriate muscular tension simply to try to fix and sustain this position. Far from its original objective of allowing freedom of movement, holding a fixed, turned out starting position with muscle-led tension restricts movement, is inefficient in terms of muscular engagement and energy consumption and will undermine speed, power and stamina. If we make the slightest shift of the attention, however, to focus on the objective of the rotation (EF), and we imagine a continuous outward rotation or spiraling intention that never arrives, then the lower body is energized, mobile and ready for any movement eventuality. The rotation is sustained by this mind-led intention and minimum muscular effort (jin).

Imagine sending energy down directly from the lower-body energy centre and allow it to spiral outwards, equally around each limb. Guide the energy in a continuous motion across the thighs, wrapping around and spiraling outwards across the inside of the knee and the calf and again across the inside of the ankle joint and foot and onwards down into the earth (figure 4.2). When spontaneously introduced into company class for the first time, ballet master Javier Torres notices that this shift of attention has an immediate impact that reenergizes the professional dancer's use of turnout to reintegrate the action into the global movement intention (Torres 2019).

If the idea of guiding *actual* energy spiraling down into the earth is not for you, then there are a multitude of tangible or imaginary spiraling foci that you might choose from to achieve the same movement effect of the turnout (figure 2.3 and table 6.1). If we consider this from an Eastern movement perspective – *where the mind goes . . . blood and energy follow* (Quian 2017) – then *any* EF you choose that inspires the desired movement outcome, whether spiraling object or metaphorical image, will act as a guide for the mind and will direct energy flow. It could be practiced, for example, with teaching resources such as tape or a resistance band or by imagining a coloured spiraling line, a child's spinning toy or the opposing movement of two tornados. I'm sure you have your own creative EF ideas for focusing on the movement objective that are appropriate in your dance context.

PARALLEL

As with the concept of the synergistic opposites yin and yang in Eastern movement, it's important to balance our practice and to respect the converse of any desired movement intention. This is also true with posture and the relationship of turnout to parallel. Dancing with an outward rotation, or turnout, of the legs *all* of the time is not the most effective way to develop the desired rotation nor build the required strength to achieve the posture's intention. Parallel position cannot simply be seen as the absence of turnout, as it is sometimes seen in dance. Parallel position, as the yin complementing

Attention and Focus in Practice

TURNOUT – USING THE SPIRAL

Javier Torres, international teacher, choreographer, former professional dancer

In tendu to the back, most people forget this spiral, and they miss the proper work on the en dehors and literally pull the weight back because the spiral gives in. When the spiral really works, in the right direction, immediately your weight is right. I noticed the difference in the whole company because it's a change of approach, a new way of using my language, and it really gives results very quickly. It's very concrete, not an imaginary picture, and it's still concentrated on the turnout and takes the focus to where you are standing. When you think of the spiral, you're already looking for a direction and you're going away, out, external.

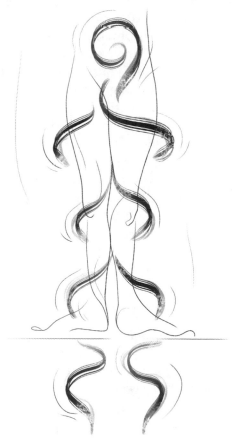

Figure 4.2   Turnout spiral – the continuous intention of the outward rotation.

the yang of turnout, is respected and sustained with attention to the two-way flow of energy (see figure 4.1) and to the active space created between the parallel leg lines.

Approaching both the outward rotation and the parallel stance as continuous movement intentions, whilst allowing space and 'breathing' joints in the lower body, means that both of these preparatory stances provide energized, active starting points with the body poised for any movement eventuality. These fluid postures then permit us to introduce a practice of continual renewal of energy as we dance because the chain reaction promotes a 'breathing' rather than a 'closed' sacrum area and a spacious rather than a rigid spine. See exploration 5.4a.

PORT DE BRAS

The original objective of the port de bras, according to Eastern movement practice, is to gather, give, lift and lower energy through the body. Ports de bras energize our movements and communicate our movement intentions beyond the confines of our own physical body, connecting us with other human beings and to the shared universal energy field. The logic of port de bras is beautiful and profound and is constructed around the principal energy centres in the body and the energy meridians than run from the vital organs and radiate out through the extremities like an intricate stellar system. It is perhaps the clearest physical embodiment of our binary universe: endlessly expanding, gathering, containing, lifting, expulsing, giving, extending, lowering, expanding and gathering energy in a binary cycle of gather and give. A return to these original objectives represents a source of inspiration, an ideal EF and a cohesion of upper-body movement quality.

Let's do a simple demi and full port de bras and take your attention to these inspirational, potential connections. Chi kung suggests we 'play' with our movement rather than 'working' at our movement, so choose your favourite slow music to accompany you and play with the energy.

EXPLORATION 4.1 – GATHER-AND-GIVE CYCLE OF PORT DE BRAS

Standing in a natural first position or open parallel, bring your attention first to the movement of the surrounding air, oxygen and energy field. Allow air and energy to circulate around and through you, creating space within. With 'breathing' joints, allow the head to float on the rising energy.

4.1(a) – Preparatory 'Breathing' Arm

Make a large circle with the arms (or take a classical bras bas position) and embrace the energy circling in and around the lower body. Expand and allow breath in and widen the circle to capture fresh energy from the energy field and replenish the body.

Gather and draw energy into the lower-body energy centre (dan tien or classical bras bas position). The preparatory breathing arm allows us to bring the attention into the present moment, quiet the mind and signal to the body that all is calm and well. See figure 4.3.

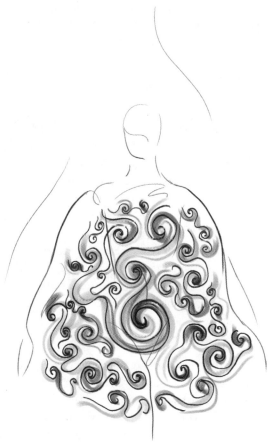

Figure 4.3   Gather and draw energy into the lower-body energy centre – dan tien or classical bras bas position.

4.1(b) – Half or Demi Port de Bras

The encircled bras bas space contains billions of dancing energy molecules that spiral in and around the power centre of the lower body (Myss 1998) like glorious champagne bubbles, enlivening and lighting up the body and the organs. Press the breath out and lift the armful of dancing energy molecules upwards towards the solar plexus and the heart energy centre (classical first position); expand and allow breath in as you arrive. Allow the position to rest on the rising, spiraling energy without tension. Breathe naturally and suspend there a moment.

Bring your attention to rest on the connection between the energy of the solar plexus, quite literally the sun of our energetic star system (centre of the self: self-understanding, self-esteem, self-confidence) and the heart energy centre (the emotional

(continued)

centre that mediates between the physical and the spiritual, the universal) (Myss 1998). Sense the energy circling through the solar plexus and the heart centre, coursing around the circle, leaping across the void between the hands and fingers, connecting and continuing, and gathering electrical charge like a vortex (see figure 3.4).

When you are ready, expand and allow breath in. The 'potential' breath activates and lifts the position. With your out-breath, slowly release the vortexing energy molecules outwards. Let the hands distance themselves one from another as you slowly make space to release the molecules. Sense the connecting, stretching threads of honey-like energy between the fingertips as they separate. Return the dancing energy molecules to the universal energy field. Energy meridians from the heart descend the insides of the arms and hands to send our intention and energy out through the pericardium or heart protector meridian (through our middle fingers) and through the heart meridian (through the little finger) (Wright 2001). Energy molecules will stick a little like static to you and your human energy field, so take your time to release them all until the circle is almost wide open to the sides (second position). Thank them for dancing with you and send the energy molecules back into the energy field or to other partner dancers or to distant observers.

Activate the second position by allowing breath in, turn and begin to lower and gather fresh energy molecules from the energy field (figure 4.3). Breathing, draw them into the lower-body power centre and embrace the sphere of moving energy that is extending through and around the body. The arms are full of energy and ready to cycle or circle again.

4.1(c) – Full Port de Bras

With the sustained out-breath, guide and lift the circling energy up through the body. Sense it swirling around, behind and through the spine and lighting up the lower-body organs as it passes. With the in-breath, connect again with the energy of the solar plexus and the heart. This time press the breath out and guide the dancing energy upwards like an inner smile rising past the delicate organs of the nervous system. Let it stroke across the face and brain to connect with the crown energy, which is the centre of our higher consciousness and spirit and direct connection with the universe (fifth position, or couronne) (Myss 1998). Breathe naturally and suspend there a moment, making space for the golden energy circling and dancing around the crown.

Bring your attention to the connection between the energy of the crown, our higher thoughts and the larger universe. Let your fingertips play in the stream of energy coming from the crown and connecting you onwards and upwards.

When you are ready, expand and allow breath in, and as you breathe out, slowly stretch and separate the connection between the fingertips and the hands and release the energy molecules out into the universe from the crown. They flow through the middle finger (pericardium meridian) and the little finger (heart meridian) and back into the universe, charged and coloured by your unique energetic intention. Thank them for playing with you as you watch them dancing off towards the heavens (figure 4.4).

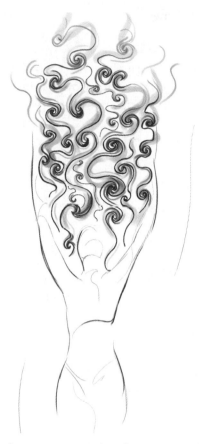

Figure 4.4   Give and release energy molecules out into the universe from the crown energy centre – fifth position, or couronne.

Take your time to release them all until the curve of the arms is wide to the sides (second position). Reactivate the second position by allowing breath in, suspend and turn to gather fresh energy molecules again from the energy field and draw them and store them in the lower-body power centre (figure 4.3). Suspend there a moment and breathe naturally. The arms surround the power centre of the body and are full of energy and ready to dance.

Before you move on, notice the sensations in your body. What are you feeling? Do you feel lighter? Supported? Buoyant? Do you feel increased energy flowing within and around the body? How did the quality differ from your habitual port de bras? Did the port de bras feel more consequential, more substantial? Take a moment to jot down any creative ideas, sensations or connections that resonated with you as you attended to these energy foci.

Did you notice that the two energy meridians that radiate out through the upper body from the heart centre send energy through the port de bras and out via the middle and little fingers? This corresponds with the emphasis placed in the classical hand position. Is this a coincidence? Is it significant, do you think?

Attending to the flow of energy through the port de bras promotes a strong, fluid and expansive movement and a sense of substantial arms that is often missing in practice. It provides a perfect external focus and restores the port de bras to its original, vital significance. It replenishes energy throughout our dancing and facilitates stamina, staying power and sensitive communication.

We took quite a few breath cycles to complete our port de bras in exploration 4.1 so that we could pay attention to all the connections and sensations. A flowing port de bras, however, might use as few as four breaths (figure 4.5). Here is an example:

- In to contain and lift
- Out to give and extend
- In to transition or turn
- Out to lower and gather energy in the lower body

All combinations of port de bras follow the binary gather-and-give cycle, lifting and moving energy clearly between the lower, heart and crown energy centres and propelling it through the extension of the limbs and beyond through our movement. The connecting threads of energy stretch and trail as hands and arms separate one from another, remaining for some distance as we transition from positions such as first to fourth or from fifth couronne to give energy out in an arabesque line, for example (see figure 3.4). Each imaginable combination has us gather, contain, lift, give and lower energy, drawing it inwards towards the body, arms full and ready to go.

In exploration 4.1, I proposed a typical breath cycle to support the flow of energy; however, the breath can be coordinated in whatever way feels most appropriate to you, to the choreography or to the dance context. Energy can also be guided through our system and beyond with just the mind, the intention and our attention without the support of the coordinated breath.

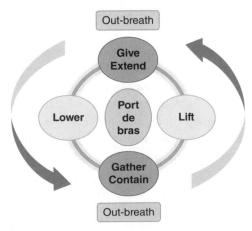

Figure 4.5   The gather-and-give cycle of port de bras.

Chi kung practice reminds us not to become too dependent or attached to a particular way of using the breath to move energy that might simply become another movement habit. Leading with the mind, our intention and attention ensures that we remain 100 per cent in the present and gives us the freedom to revisit our dance with fresh eyes.

For explorations to enhance energy sensing in port de bras, revisit explorations 3.6*a*, 3.6*b* and 3.8. See exploration 5.2 to develop the lower-body power centre as a constant energy source throughout your dancing.

If moving and connecting with universal energy does not work in your dance context, then choose from the myriad EF sensory and imaginary ideas in figure 2.3. You might choose the mental rehearsal of seeing the desired movement path and shapes in space, working with sensory metaphoric images like embracing clouds or sending coloured lines or lasers out into space from the extensions, or simply to experience the proprioceptive feeling of the two-way or five-way pull of the extended movement. Port de bras is a gift to work with as we explore different EF possibilities. We seem less tempted to consciously control the limbs in these upper-body movements, and any EF approach you choose will promote the benefits outlined in table 2.2, because *where the mind will go, blood and energy will follow* (Quian 2017).

THE EXTENDED LEG – TENDU

Imagine for a moment that the open and 'breathing' quality of the arms, hands and upper body during port de bras might be transferable to the movement of the legs, feet and lower body. Might it be possible to work with breathing joints *despite* a focus on support and strength? Perhaps it's imperative to work with a fluid quality and breathing joints, as Eastern movement practice suggests, precisely *because* the demands are support, stability and strength. Could the extension of the feet and ankles feel like the port de bras hands and breathing wrists, guiding energy spiraling through the movement and beyond as an extension of the movement intention?

EXPLORATION 4.2 – SENSING CONSTRICTED ENERGY

Let's try a typical more-is-more approach that we might adopt with the lower body and use it in upper-body movement a moment so that we can experience what happens to energy flow when we use a more-is-more approach. Let's take a port de bras position with the same approach of maximum effort that we might use for the extended leg and pointed foot. Throw your arms wide into a beautiful expansive second position and let's engage lots of muscles: grip or scrunch your fingers tight in a fixed classical hand position as you might do with a pointed foot. Hold and close off the flow of energy through the wrist joint as you might do with the ankle, and similarly maintain and fix the shoulder position, as you might do to control the turn-out at the hip. Sustain that position for a few moments and notice what's happening

(continued)

EXPLORATION 4.2 (continued)

to the flow of energy. What's happening in your body? Observe your sensations, and when you *can't* sustain the position any longer, drop your arms and shake out.

What did you notice? Did you forget to breathe? Did the action become heavy? Did your temperature increase? Perhaps you began to sweat or your arms began to tremble even. How long could you have sustained your second position? Could you sense the energy constricted within the position?

Rather than freely flowing out as an extension of the line, blocked, constricted energy provokes increased muscular tension that creeps back up the chain inwards towards the centre, towards the shoulders, neck and even face muscles, in this case. With no exit route, energy will turn incessantly in turmoil. It starts to overheat or burn in the constricted muscles, which creates the aching or burning sensation that you might experience when trying to hold a position (West 1997). The same happens with the lower body, feet, ankles, legs and hip joints. Holding or gripping results in constricted, boiling energy, and the movement becomes increasingly muscular, producing a chain reaction of inappropriate muscular engagement, unnecessary effort and slow, inconsistent movement that is easily exhausted. Power is easily depleted.

When you begin to look with fresh eyes at the lower-body movement of other dancers, you start to see this more-is-more approach. You see many blocked or closed-off ankle joints and tightly scrunched toe joints and excessive muscular effort at all dance skills levels. Despite the foot being potentially hidden away in tights or shoes, the detrimental impact of the inappropriate tension and holding to the flow of energy and the resulting inefficiency of the lower body is immediately visible and palpable.

A fresh approach is to first seek a similar 'breathing' sensation in the ankle joint as you already enjoy in the 'breathing' wrist joint of the port de bras. Allowing the ankle joint to be spacious and to breathe results in an opening of the joint and a potential increase in the range of motion, or arching line, that is one of dance's desired movement outcomes.

Just like the hands, the legs and feet are part of our stellar system of energy meridians radiating out from the centre, from individual vital organs of the lower body, down the legs and out through the ankle and toes. The energy spirals down through the legs from the lower energy centre to freely flow through the breathing joints (figure 4.2). Long, spacious toe joints, reaching like fingers, are an extension of the movement intention and guide the energy out into the universe. In Eastern therapeutic practice, therapists are taught to have hands like water that flow over the forms they touch, firm yet without tension. Perhaps feet like water – strong and powerful, yet supple and breathing – might be a beautiful and effective movement objective for dancers.

Let's take a moment to revisit the action of the whole extension of the tendu. This is a foundational skill learnt in our earliest, most formative years. Depending on the approach of our teachers, this foundational learning establishes the control approach we will take for the rest of our dancing lives. Thanks to the effect of mirror neurons (Freedman 2016), we learn movement and absorb such things as appropriate effort and breathing, mindset and approach to control directly by transmission, simply by following our first teachers. (See chapter 6 for more on teaching by transmission.)

The approach to an early tendu then informs our approach to all other, more demanding lower-limb actions yet to come. In terms of its mechanical action, a tendu is a tendu whether we are 5 years old or 50, and yet the fascinating thing about a tendu is that there must be a hundred different ways to execute the same action in terms of the desired movement effect: energy, quality, pressure and musicality of the attack and accents. So it's clear that the key to mastery of a tendu is not in the movement action itself but is in the intention and our attention to those qualities. Teachers use a multitude of diverse EF, metaphoric imagery to achieve the qualities they seek such as push down through the floor, caress the floor, trace a line, like a pizza slicer, think of the space in the dégagé (the space, the separation from centre line). The original French vocabulary – tendu meaning to stretch – provides a perfect EF and concurs with an Eastern approach by bringing our attention to the tendu action of stretching and extending. It's a verb, not a position. Just like the en dehors rotation (figure 4.2), from an Eastern perspective, a tendu would be approached as a continuous movement intention that reaches away from the lower-body energy centre by sending energy spiraling down and out through both legs and through breathing, open joints. It continues as an intention in the mind long after the physical dégagé position has been reached. The tendu then draws distant energy back up and into the lower energy centre like a wave with the closing action. Attending to this continuous movement intention and following the flow of energy out and beyond with the mind (EF) produces a different, minimal muscular engagement in the legs. It promotes a longer aesthetic line, enhanced movement quality and ease and speed of movement that paves the way for developing the technique for efficient, lighter movement and improved stamina as the demands on the lower limbs increase.

BALANCE

Consider for a moment the idea that the body is made up principally of space, energy, water and oxygen and only a very small percentage of what we might consider solid matter, as we explored in chapter 3. Space, energy, water and oxygen all follow the same universal laws of spiraling movement (figure 3.3). Whether in the massive movement of the universal elements, in the weather systems, in the oceans, in a tiny drop of water or in a human cell, there is no such thing as stillness. Energy might be blocked or constricted, but its nature moves and spirals continuously trying to find a way to flow onwards. So as hard as we might try, we cannot consciously control a balance or aim to hold a fixed position by gripping muscles. To expect our bodies to do so flies in the face of their nature. However, many dancers try constantly to resolve the conflict between the desired ideal of stability and the inevitable variability of human movement (Hopper et al. 2018).

Balance, as in the case of the expert surfer, is a dynamic action of millions of in-the-moment microadjustments to verticality. If our expectation is that our balance *should* be still, as many of us have been taught, we attempt to balance by controlling and adjusting our own body parts, and we interrupt the body's own fast, reflexive processes. By consciously trying to fix our posture, we induce a chain reaction of movement dysfunction, like the thinking cat we imagined trying to catch the fly by consciously instructing itself (see chapter 3).

For optimum balance, guide the mind with a single attentional focus on the intended movement outcome, the simpler and clearer the better (EF). That EF acts as a kind of blueprint or road map for the mind and muscles. This can be any EF of your choice; here are some examples: a real vertical line in the studio, such as a column, or the edge of the mirror, wall or window; an imaginary vertical red line going through the centre of the body and beyond; the proprioceptive sensation of the two-way vertical action of pushing the floor and reaching for the sky; the large circulation of energy (figure 4.1) or surfing on a fountain of energy (exploration 4.3).

Bring your attention to the EF and aim to filter out all other distracting information or inner dialogue. Reset and refresh the EF in your mind as often as possible throughout to help the body access its automatic control processes and to adapt and achieve the desired dynamic balance. Once dancers achieve a fast, reflexive verticality, we are often tempted to release the EF from our minds and take our attention somewhere else; however, it's important to sustain the imaginary or real EF consistently all the way to the end of the movement to ensure a secure, stable closing or conclusion. Let's experiment with the balance from the perspective of energy flow, approaching it like surfing on a fountain of energy (West 1997).

EXPLORATION 4.3 – ENERGY FOUNTAIN TO BALANCE

Before you start taking your focus to the flow of energy, establish a baseline for comparison by taking a balance in retiré as you habitually would. Use a whole-foot or demi-pointe balance with your arms in first or fifth position. Use the wall or a barre to assist your stability as you prepare. As you release and take the position, observe how your stability feels today. Can you identify the strategies you typically use? Are you using an image? A proprioceptive feeling? Are you attempting to adjust your own posture to control the stability? Are you holding your breath? Perhaps you are doing all of these. Now, release and come down. Take a few moments if you want to write down your habitual balance control process and observations from this baseline balance.

Ready to go again? Stand in a natural first or 'spiraling' fifth position, with weight firmly and evenly distributed on both sides. Allow air, energy or 'water' to flow around and through the spaces made by the body. Send fluid energy from the lower energy centre through the energy highway (the spine) and beyond to enliven the internal organs and the extremities. Allow space and breathing joints. Using the mind, draw powerful energy up from deep in the earth. You can 'see' it bright like liquid light or like a water geyser or fountain shooting up from the rock. Draw it spiraling up through the body, and allow its power to lift you up, making space. The geyser or fountain shoots forcefully through your centre line, through the spine and lifts and opens the occipital area to flow through the crown and beyond. Breathe naturally throughout. Draw energy upwards with the in-breath and expel it onwards with a powerful out-breath. Use the wall or the barre as before to support you as you prepare.

Shift your weight slowly until you feel 100 per cent of the pressure and weight on the standing side, and then peel the empty leg from the floor, drawing (the leg and foot) up spiraling into retiré with no effort (figure 4.6). Allow the position to float in the buoyant movement of the fountain. (If you want press onto demi-pointe, take a slow sustained out-breath and push the floor away to rise. The energy pressure increases with the push, gushing upward with a central thrust.) Allow the arms simply to float on the water without tension; feel the movement of the energy and the upward lift and the support. Energy shoots up and out through the crown and some cascades around you back down to earth making a full, continuous circle: powerful and uplifting through the spine and descending and releasing superficial tension as it falls to earth. Allow yourself to surf with the movement and notice the body making its myriad micro-adjustments to your verticality. If you feel unstable, resist the temptation to grip or consciously control your body. Instead, take a slow breath out and bring your attention back to the EF: the sensations, the pressure into the floor, the powerful centre of the fountain spiraling, and shooting up and beyond. Breathe naturally. Release and come down.

How did this balance feel? Were you able to breathe throughout? Were some aspect of the image or sensations more present for you than others? What were they? How much effort did you use compared to the first balance? Did your sense of stability feel different? Did you feel as though you were doing less than usual? Were you able to reset your attention when it wandered? Or did you take over consciously to adjust and fix your posture?

If dancing with a control approach that uses EF is not your usual strategy for balance, then a demi-pointe balance in retiré is perhaps a challenging task to start with. Sustaining your attention on an exter-nal focus and resisting the temptation to consciously interfere and self-adjust the balance becomes easier the more you use it. Even if your first exploration was not completely successful, did you observe any interesting differences in this first example?

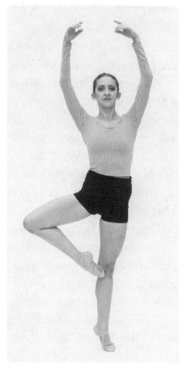

Figure 4.6   Surfing on the energy fountain, with micro-adjustments. (Kailey)

Thinking of the powerful energy fountain that you just experienced – or imagining *any* coursing water fountain – what would happen to the water flow if you tried to grasp the fountain in the middle with your hands to hold or fix the movement of the water with muscular effort? We all tried that as children with a real water fountain: The upward power of the water was dissipated and water shoots off uncontrollably at different angles and in different directions, much to our amusement. So it is too with the energy fountain; if we attempt to grip or hold the movement in the middle rather than go *with* the direction of flow, energy scatters and shoots off ineffectively at different angles. The powerful vertical trajectory is significantly diminished and fragmented, causing movement dysfunction and certain loss of balance.

The idea of sensing, interacting, 'surfing' and dancing *with* the surrounding energy (EF) rather than trying to fix and control the body (IF) *against* the natural flow of energy is a foundational concept that you can progressively experiment with and develop throughout your dance practice. This approach brings even more benefits as we move on to more complex movement combinations that require sustained power and fluidity or explosive power, precision and speed.

REVISITING COMPLEX MOVEMENT – THE SLOW SUSTAIN OF ADAGE

The demands of adage to produce fluid, balanced, seemingly effortless and yet powerful, sustained movement with a particular attention to the correct movement form and line make it perhaps the most challenging skill in dance. Adage requires stability, consistent strength and stamina, and at the same time minimal muscular engagement to produce fluid, calm and expressive movement. As we saw in the study on the attentional focus of professional dancers (Guss-West and Wulf 2016), executing an adage – balance in arabesque, for example – seems to incite the greatest tendency to interfere and attempt to consciously control our own limbs to achieve the desired line (IF). This temptation is probably the result of the combination of the amount of potential thinking time available in slow, sustained adage; the lack of an alternative supportive control strategy (EF); previous IF teaching feedback; and the performance pressure and anxiety to achieve a certain movement form or line. Satisfyingly, just the small shift of attention prompted by introducing an EF control approach results in a marked difference in the quality and the effort of this complex combination of movement objectives. Immediate benefits are experienced and observed by the dancer and teacher alike. Let's revisit some of the component parts of adage using several examples of external attention and mind-led strategies that promote a global movement cohesion and facilitate these technical demands.

THE EXTENDED LEG – DEVELOPPÉ

As with the tendu, the movement intention of the developpé is a continuous, unfolding journey as its name in French suggests, never arriving at a fixed end point, going beyond with the attention long after the desired physical position might be attained. To achieve the necessary, seemingly contradictory qualities of the fluid, light, high extension with powerful sustain, we might use a mind-led Eastern approach. We can focus the attention in the same way we did for the powerful, less-is-more arm press (exploration 3.7) to achieve these fish-like qualities. Even though we may have done thousands of developpés in our dancing life, aim to approach the movements today *as if* for the very first time, with a clear mind that is 100 per cent in the present moment.

EXPLORATION 4.4 – EXTENDED LEG – DEVELOPPÉ

Standing in a natural first position, drop your breathing down towards the lower energy centre and bring your attention to the sensations in the body and to the energy and air circling around and through the spaces created by your body. Embrace the circling energy of the lower energy centre or take a fluid bras bas and allow energy to ascend, circling up through the spine, floating the head, lengthening the occipital bone. Allow energy to escape beyond your physical body.

   With joints melting, sink into the ocean of energy and oxygen surrounding you and slowly shift your weight until it is 100 per cent on one side. During the fondu, one side is 'full' of pressure and is the full, or working, side. The other side is the 'empty', or 'playing', side. With an in-breath, draw the energy of the port de bras and the empty leg, spiraling up to the knee to retiré. Feel the touch and the pressure of your dance shoe, sock or the 'empty' foot as it traces the line against your supporting side. Breathe naturally and suspend a moment with energy circling through and around the heart and solar plexus centres (first position). Before you move on, imagine clearly where you will direct the energy of the extending 'empty' leg. What does the movement line look like? What is the angle? Is it out to the trees? Up to the stars? Keep that energy trajectory clear in your mind, perhaps give it a colour or a quality. Empty the leg of tension, ready to direct the energy flow, and reactivate your retiré and first position as you expand and allow breath in. With a slow, sustained out-breath, open the port de bras from the heart and unfold the playing leg. Send energy continually spiraling out through the unfolding developpé so that it follows your imaginary line (figure 4.7). Keep it clear in your mind . . . empty . . . outwards . . . no tension. Let the leg and joints simply act as an empty conduit so that maximum energy can flow. Guide the energy spiraling out through breathing joints, through the extension. Breathe naturally, and send your energy out . . . out . . . out . . . never arriving . . . as far as you can imagine.

   Expand and allow breath in to support the lowering of the empty leg and port de bras. Gather fresh energy as they lower. The standing side pushes down into the earth to increase the pressure, sending energy up through the body. Push to straighten

(continued)

drawing energy back into the lower-body energy centre. Notice that the weight is evenly on both sides as energy circulates through the body. Embrace the energy in the lower body (bras bas). Breathe naturally and relax.

What sensations did you observe in your body? How did it compare to your habitual approach? How much effort were you using? Were you breathing throughout? Could you have sustained longer? How big did your movement feel? What was the quality of the movement? Was it solid? Fluid? Shaky? Constant? Jot down a few key words to describe the immediate sensations so that you can consolidate the new learning for the body and brain.

Take your time and do this exercise again on the other side as slowly as on the first side. Bring your attention to this moment and be 100 per cent present. It takes time to register and embody new proprioceptive sensations. It takes time to override habitual patterns of thought and their associated effort that you've recorded so many times before. Take your attention to this moment and this space, and the proprioceptive sensations will be imprinted effectively. The more you shift your attention to attend to these sensations, the more accessible they will become when you want to apply them in faster, more demanding movement challenges.

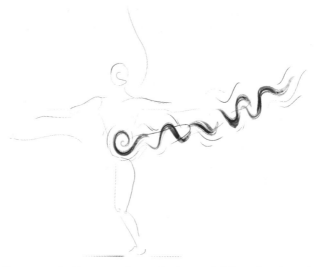

Figure 4.7   Energy spiraling out through the unfolding developpé.

ARABESQUE – FIVE SIMULTANEOUS DIRECTIONS OF ENERGY

Continuing from a focus on a single extension using mind-led energy, let's take a look at the sublime arabesque. The origin of the French ballet term refers to the innovative curves of early Middle-Eastern architecture: 'An ornamental design consisting of intertwined flowing lines' (Lexico 2017). Observed from the outside, the arabesque in Western dance might look like a fixed position comprising a series of angles and straight lines; however, when dancing we can experience our arabesque from the perspective of its original movement intention, as a series of continuous flowing curves. Just as we experienced in previous explorations for tendu and developpé, if we shift our attention to the *continuous* aspect of the movement intention (EF), our arabesque takes on new life, new dimensions, fluidity and ease.

The arabesque balance demands a complex combination of qualities: calm balance, stability and power and at the same time sensitive, expressive, breathing, flowing lines. If our expectation is to hold a fixed arabesque position rather than to surf the energy flow and adapt to the natural movement variability of the human body, then, as we saw with the balance, we disrupt the body's reflex to microadjust and achieve this complex combination of seemingly contradictory qualities. If we are tempted, even for a millisecond, to shift our attention onto an individual body part in a desire to consciously adjust the line of the arabesque (IF) rather than sustain the chosen EF, then stability will be immediately compromised, power diminished and extension limited. We withdraw energy from the whole and send the attention, *blood and energy* only into the fragmented part.

A foundational approach then to guiding the attention and enabling all of the desired qualities is to attend to the flow of energy throughout the whole system at all times. Attending to the whole system means having an holistic vision of the intention of the whole movement rather than just a partial vision – only on the height of the playing leg or only on the angle of the back, for example. A whole vision projects energy out simultaneously through the five directions equally: from the lower energy centre downwards to respect the standing side and its powerful connection to the earth, and to flow freely out through the line of the playing leg; from the heart and solar plexus energy centres out through the heart meridian fingers and beyond; and via the crown energy centre upwards and out into the universe to stabilize the five-way pull (figure 4.8). The arabesque expands from the centre outwards like an amazing radiant star or exploding firework.

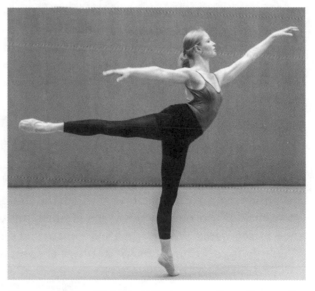

Figure 4.8   Five simultaneous directions of energy in arabesque. (Emmi)

To identify the proprioceptive sensations of this simultaneous expansion, let's start with the preparation. There's no need to extend into a high arabesque for now; the idea initially is to capture the sensations of the movement initiation and the energy flow in this concept. The challenge is to attend to the curve and to simultaneously send out energy in all five directions equally. This whole vision promotes the stability, power, expansive fluidity and expression of the movement.

EXPLORATION 4.5(a) – THE FIVE SIMULTANEOUS DIRECTIONS OF ENERGY – ARABESQUE

Prepare a full standing side and extend the empty, or playing, leg of your choice behind in a dégagé à terre, and take a moment to identify the five directions of pull. Give a little press or extension out in each direction that will become the arabesque, one after another to refresh and enliven them all. Allow energy to flow through and around the shapes made by your body and give space for the joints to breathe. Relax and lower the arms.

Prepare the port de bras as you did before, gathering energy and drawing it up to the solar plexus and heart centres (first position). Suspend and breathe naturally. Expand and allow breath in preparation. Taking a slow out-breath, press down and extend out, releasing energy downwards, outwards and upwards from the lower, the heart, and the crown energy centres. Expand and grow a few centimetres in all five directions equally in a glorious, generous curve.

Experiment with the five-way, simultaneous initiation a couple of times. It might take a few tries to identify parts that are initiating separately and any microdelays between each of the five directions that might be occurring. Take your attention to the coordination of the sustained, powerful out-breath; the push down and out; and the five-way extension until it ignites as one. You might think of it like the action of striking a match – we coordinate the preparatory action of the hand in a curve that presses and pushes away until it ignites, sparking in all directions. Take a moment to note any creative thoughts or images that came to you as you were exploring that five-way expansion or anything you observed about your own habitual arabesque initiation.

If you look, you can frequently observe dancers initiating arabesque in a series of body-part steps with a microdelay between each initiation. This might be typically first one arm, then the next, then the playing leg, then perhaps the connection to the ground and finally the crown. Given the movement variability of the human body, it's challenging to achieve this dynamic balance in segments. When instability ensues, it's often because one direction of energy is too dominant, or another is completely absent from the mind.

As you practice observing others, your ability to 'see' their lines of extending energy will develop and your ability to identify when and where energy is closed off or not flowing. (See exploration 6.1 for teaching ideas to encourage the simultaneous five-way extension of the arabesque.)

Once the preparation ignites as one whole movement, like the striking of a match, then the arabesque continues to power outwards and upwards into space in the five directions of trajectory on the initial, sustained out-breath. The principles of mind-led energy flow mean that the attention to the five directions and the intention of the flow continue long after maximum physical possibilities have been surpassed, beyond until there is no breath left. We can easily suspend a moment in space with nothing – no breath – just outward flowing energy and space. If it's a very long, slow arabesque curve, then expansion and renewed in-breath continue throughout the extension, powering out further with each out-breath. In the flow of choreography, the transitional in-breath happens naturally as a reflex action, ideally coordinated to support the lowering from arabesque on the incoming breath and energy. The lowering movement gathers and draws energy into the lower energy centre in preparation for the next power-out movement (the next powerful, outward, highlight or yang moment of a movement coordinated on an out-breath).

Perhaps the choreography demands a further sustained power-out movement into fondu, demi-pointe rise, suspension or penché (tilting), for instance. Continuing, we expand, replenish and allow breath in (allongé) and initiate the next movement intention clearly with the mind and press outwards and onwards with the breath.

EXPLORATION 4.5(b) – CONTINUING THE ARABESQUE – PENCHÉ

To lead the arabesque curve into penché, for example, refresh all of the attentional foci of the arabesque before initiating the movement: See or sense the five equal directions and the energy spiraling down the standing side, respecting its connection to the earth and yet radiating energy outwards in all directions (figure 4.9a). With an in-breath, trace a distant curve to initiate the incline. The in-breath expansion supports the transition and the displacement of weight. Float forwards on the expansion and the breath and send energy in all directions in long, swooping diagonal curves, like the trail of a shooting star, until you connect in your mind between the earth and stars (figure 4.9b). Use a slow sustained out-breath to reach between the polarities, sensing the powerful magnetic pull between the earth and the universe. The EF distance effect brings increased power and sustain to your movement (see figure 3.6) (Wulf 2013). To support the transition, expand and allow breath in and retrace the five distant curves and send breath powerfully out as you recover verticality.

(continued)

EXPLORATION 4.5(b) *(continued)*

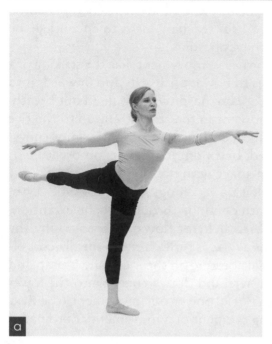 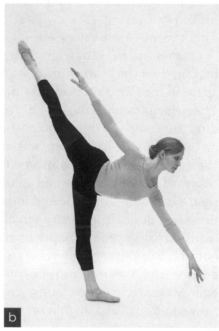

Figure 4.9   Distance effect – (*a*) the five directions of the arabesque reach as one (*b*) to penché to earth and stars. (Emmi)

The choice of out- or in-breath to best support the demands of a movement is of course a personal choice, and you can experiment with coordinating breath and energy flow and decide which you feel supports the desired quality and expression of a particular choreography. Calm, coordinated, flowing breath brings innumerable physiological and neurological benefits (Liponis 2007). Use your preferred coordination to guide the energy. Not breathing, however, as dancers so often do in challenging moments, is not an option!

ATTITUDE – A GLORIOUS CIRCLING ORBIT

If we approach an attitude *as if* for the very first time, with fresh eyes, we might see a beautiful, arcing suspension of continuous, circling energy that surrounds the human body like a golden orbit. With familiarity, it's tempting to pay less attention to its circling movement intention and try to fix and hold the attitude or control the desired form with muscle-led effort (li energy, IF). When we initiate an attitude with an IF control approach, however, limbs are held and foreshortened, and the shape becomes fragmented, simply a series of individual angular, body parts. The sense of the cohesive, expressive, flowing movement is lost.

EXPLORATION 4.6 – ATTITUDE – A GLORIOUS CIRCLING ORBIT

Suspend any disbelief you may have, and let's defamiliarize ourselves and take a fresh look at an attitude. Expand, make space and breathe as you have done in previous preparations. Gather fresh energy into the lower energy centre. Send spiraling energy en dehors into the earth, connecting and respecting the standing side. Substantial, revolving energy in the lower energy centre, or power centre, rises and suspends the upper body, extending it towards the universe. Sense the powerful, supporting two-way pull of the earth and the universe. Distance the 'playing' side (top arm and gesture leg) from the standing side, making space and curving far away from centre. Allow the standing side to breathe. Continuous energy flows from the lower energy centre, through the heart centre, through the top arm and out through the fingers. The energy jumps the void between the top fingertips (fourth position) and the 'playing' foot, like arcing electricity, to connect powerfully through the gesture curve and continue onwards and upwards in a golden orbit of continuous motion. Feel the energy orbiting the body, buoyant and suspending it in space between earth and universe. Sense the dancing energy within the orbit, filling the space made by the arc of the body (figure 4.10). Feel the generous circle of energy as it embraces and curves around the space. 'Surf' with the circling energy a moment and see clearly the two separate movement intentions: the verticality of the two-way pull between earth and stars on the standing side and the dazzling, orbiting energy of the playing side. Place your attention in the generous space created. Embrace and curve around the space as you catch dancing energy in your attitude circle.

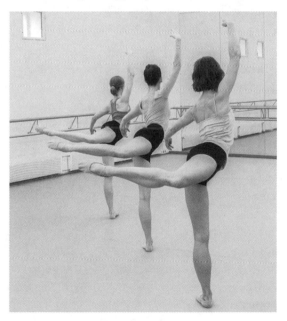

Figure 4.10   The circling energy of the attitude, suspended between earth and stars. (Emmi, Kailey and Tehri)

If guiding and connecting energy to the surrounding energy field in explorations 4.5 and 4.6 seems intangible or inaccessible as your chosen control approach, there are plenty of alternative real, sensory and imaginary EF that can be adopted. Perhaps start by introducing a proximal EF in the arabesque such as sensing the pressure of the floor or imagining the five directions reaching out into space. Or you can choose from any number of metaphoric images. Choose images for the supplementary information they promote such as a suggested form, dynamic or quality – for example, an exploding firework or star might promote a brief, yet expansive, arabesque, or a more earthly, majestic oak tree with deep roots and reaching branches might promote a sustained, stable arabesque (figure 4.11). For an attitude, you might, for example, focus clearly on just the circle created by the top arm and attitude leg. Any appropriate image of your choice will guide the mind and focus the attention and send energy, oxygen and nutrients in the direction of the intention: *where the mind will go, blood and energy will follow* (Quian 2017). There is always the option to experiment with a progressively distant external focus later. The distance effect increases the physical benefits of stability, consistency, optimum energy and minimum muscular engagement, improving stamina. The mental benefits that result from the free cognitive reserve are also further enhanced such as improved management of performance stress and anxiety and heightened artistic listening and expression. In Eastern movement practice, we learn to progressively harness the benefits of this distance effect to intensify the energy, oxygen and nutrients sent to the extremities. We take advantage of the two-way, magnetic-like pull of earth and universe to stabilize the movement (figure 4.1). Then by sending energy further with the mind and continuously drawing it back into our

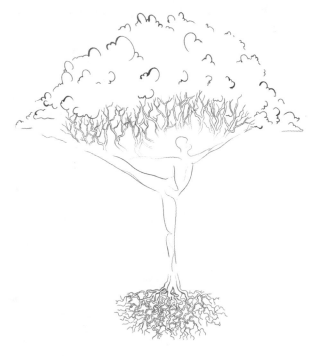

Figure 4.11   A metaphorical image of a majestic oak tree with deep roots and reaching branches to promote stability and sustain in arabesque.

lower energy centre, we charge the surrounding energy field. This increases the volume of the flow of energy through our movements and develops our capacity to direct energy. The energy field surrounding us becomes condensed and compact, enhancing powerful, effective movement.

ROND DE JAMBE – ATTENTION TO THE WHOLE

Let's take a look at a more complex, sustained adage movement: rond de jambe en l'air (a curve of the leg in the air). This movement can feel extremely heavy and muscle led unless we adopt an EF approach and take our attention to the coordination of the whole rather than the parts. The principle of the full leg and the empty, or playing, leg is particularly effective when applied to this action.

Prepare by expanding, gathering and respecting the standing side as you have done for other explorations. Send energy spiraling out of the unfolding, empty or playing extension from the lower energy centre to a distant focal point, either in the studio or beyond, as you practiced with the extended leg – developpé (exploration 4.4). The slow, sustained, outward flow of energy now traces a smooth, golden arc around the room, cutting through the space like a laser or like the beam from a lighthouse. Coordinated breathing facilitates the fluidity and the renewal of energy throughout the action. You might use a sustained out-breath as you extend energy forwards, out and around. As you trace your arc toward the side to second, for example, expand and allow breath in and the joints to breathe. This expansion and influx of energy and oxygen lifts and suspends us in space, easing the transition and the smooth rotation around from the side (second) to behind. Complete the arc with the slow, sustained out-breath to its conclusion in the arabesque line, extending until you have almost no breath left. Send energy out continuously through the line, suspending with nothing. The in-breath will surely replenish itself as a reflex action as soon as you change the movement intention to lower, gather in and transition into the next movement.

Because this is potentially a strenuous movement, the temptation is to have just a partial vision of the rond de jambe and see it only as a lower-limb action. If you focus only on the action of the playing leg, however, you sacrifice power and stability in the whole. Seeing the movement as a whole, in its three dimensions, and attending clearly to the synchronization of and relationship between the moving port de bras and the trajectory of the playing leg ensures the benefits of an EF and maintains energy in the whole system throughout the action. In figure 4.12a, you see dancer Tehri prepare by bringing her attention to two touch points and their relationship to one another. She keeps the two touch points in her mind as she guides the arc of the movement and attends to the constantly changing relationship between the two. See figures 4.12*b-d*. Focusing on the pull of the two touch points creates connecting threads of energy between them. The moving elements are in continuous coordination like the parts of a gyroscope moving as one whole to produce a cohesive, captivating movement.

Just as with the port de bras, when we extend outwards from a position that contains energy (bras bas, first, fifth), the energy stretches, arcing between the distancing hands, fingers and feet (see figure 3.4). This energy phenomenon occurs with any of the body's extensions, so, similarly, it occurs between the extensions and relationship of arms and upper-body movements and the legs and lower-body actions. Extensions move through space leaving a wake of waves in the energy field, like passing boats moving across water.

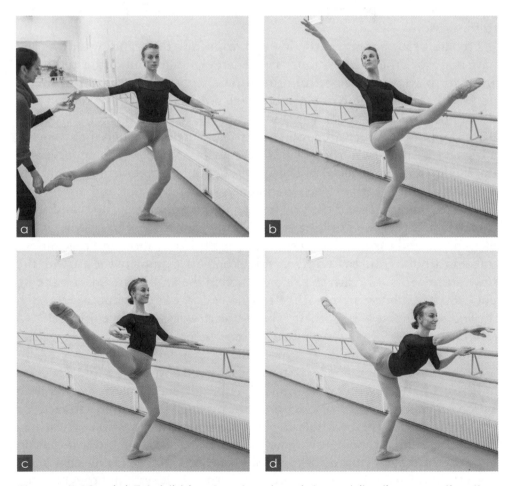

Figure 4.12   *(a)* Establishing two touch points and *(b-d)* connecting the energy threads by focusing on the changing relationship of the points. (Clare and Tehri)

FONDU AND TEMPS LIÉ

The exquisite slow, sustained movement of adage is not a series of individual movements and positions but a continuum of movement. We pass through a series of highlights and power-out moments; however, mastering the connecting transitions (temps lié) is equally important in order to achieve the desired quality, sustain, stability and expressiveness of the whole. These transitions are also key to replenishing the energy and breath and have the function of counterbalancing all the demanding yang, power-out moments of Western dance styles. Respecting the connections and the transitions and bringing attention to their movement objectives takes our dancing to another level of power and artistry.

> It is in these controlled transitions that the lyrical beauty of adage achieves its greatest poetic power. (Ryman 2008, 77)

So let's analyse a more complex example of that continuum and flow. We'll coordinate and move through a power-out extension, moving onwards through a transitional fondu (melting) to a power-out, demi-pointe press, rise and balance in retiré and move back through a supporting fondu so that we can look at all of the connections and relationships we have explored so far. The full gather–lift–give–lower continuum never stops expanding and filling (yin) or contracting and extending out (yang) in our binary, universal movement pattern like a glorious medusa or jellyfish travelling through the wide ocean.

EXPLORATION 4.7 – THE GATHER-AND-GIVE CYCLE OF ADAGE

Start in a relaxed fifth position. Spiraling into the ground, bring your attention for a moment to the energy and air circling around you and through the spaces created by your body. Take a moment to refresh the large circulation of energy (figure 4.1). Draw earth energy up the front of the legs, through the lower energy centre and onwards, allowing the energy to powerfully lift the spine through to the universe. Draw universal energy down, stroking across the face, the front of the body, through the lower energy centre and on down the back of the legs to connect you to the earth.

With a preparatory port de bras, gather and embrace the energy of the lower energy centre (bras bas). Ascending energy circles upwards and suspends the upper body, elevates the occipital bone and escapes through the crown and beyond.

- **Prepare:** As one movement, press into the floor with the out-breath, lift energy up and out with the port de bras and separate and send energy spiraling down to extend the playing leg to the side à terre.

- **Fondu:** Expand the 'energy highway' (the spine) and make space. Allow breath in to fill the joints and the sacrum and open the occipital area. Draw in the empty leg to transition through fondu, supported by the incoming breath and energy. Lower the port de bras to gather and contain.

(continued)

EXPLORATION 4.7 *(continued)*

- **Extension:** With a sustained out-breath, push down into the earth. As the counterenergy pressure increases and ascends, unfold and send out energy in five clear directions. The mind and the attention focus on the five simultaneous directions, guiding their desired pathways, to the point of no breath.

- **Fondu:** Expand and allow breath to flood in. Create maximum space as you envelop the incoming air and energy as before. The empty leg suspends on the incoming energy in fondu position as you gather in with the lowering port de bras.

- **Rise to retiré:** With one long, sustained out-breath, push spiraling energy down into the earth, and draw the rising counterenergy upwards with the port de bras. The empty leg rides with the rising energy and suspends, with breathing joints, in retiré. Feel the light pressure and touch of the retiré against the standing side. The port de bras draws the energy up through the heart centre in an energy fountain to the crown and beyond and back out into the universe. The mind and attention focus on the two simultaneous directions – towards the earth and towards the stars – extending through to a suspension with no breath.

- **Fondu:** Expand and open, and allow breath to flood in. Lowering, embracing, gathering and containing energy in the supporting fondu transition, and so on in a beautiful, self-sustaining continuum of energy (figure 4.13).

Take a moment to jot down thoughts or sensations that came up as you focused on the continuous gather–lift–give–lower continuum for the first time. There were a lot of ideas to focus on; however, did you notice different sensations as you transitioned through fondu with this reverse, replenishing breathing? Was it more stable? More energized? How was the movement quality? Lighter? Heavier? Something else? And your stamina, could you have kept going easily?

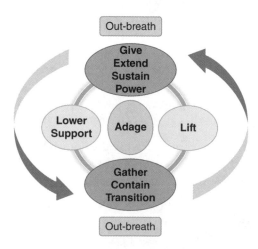

Figure 4.13   The gather-and-give cycle of adage.

The wisdom of the Eastern movement approach suggests that it is counter-productive to focus only on the highpoints in a movement phrase. If we focus on arriving rather than pay attention to the whole journey, we will soon be exhausted, and the movements will be inconsistent and unstable. The key is to flow continuously, not imagining that we have arrived at an end point or that we could *hold* a movement against the inevitable flow of energy, oxygen and water. Focusing equally on the quality and the objective of the transitions and connections (yin) supports and provides stability through challenging transfers of weight. It replenishes energy, assures continued power and stamina, and

Attention and Focus in Practice

ADAGIO – IT'S A FEELING, NOT A THOUGHT PROCESS

Stephanie Saland, dance educator and coach, former principal dancer at the New York City Ballet

I entered focused ballet training at the age of 14-1/2 years, which was considered quite a late start. Within 3-1/2 years I was in the company. Having missed fundamental training, I learned by observing and imitating my peers and was able to approximate movement until it became a reasonable facsimile of the steps. I discovered an innate inclination for adagio with its sensibility in relationship to breath and time. It allows for a feeling of control blended with yielding. I enjoyed the sculpting and shaping a body in space . . . this unfolding, unfurling, elongating, this revealing of very discrete parts of the body.

It was a feeling, not a thought process. Imagination sets in where I can have restraint and then dissemble it, mess with it! There is an aspect that feels cocreative: You can initiate a step or ignite it a certain way. You can give it a certain quality of closing and landing. Ask how ample or how far or how deep – or how you might contain yourself so you can save it for later. It's about being extremely deliberate.

I love Gelsey's [Kirkland] explanation of rotation as 'the underbelly of the body'. In class, I often tease and playfully suggest an image with young students: If you see a dog on its back, legs in the air suggesting 'pet me' – that's an image that can translate to our perception of rotation as it relates to vulnerability. So, if we flip over, we expose the underbelly – all the soft tissue and inseams as it were – the abdomen, forearms, the under arms and armpits, the throat and neck, the inner thighs. This exposing of oneself helps to bypass any sense of guarding or armor. There is a nuanced vulnerability in bringing the inner body to the frontal plane. To my mind, this encourages a quality of interiority and sincerity that translates for both dancer and audience as genuine and universal.

enhances artistic expression. (Further information about replenishing energy in motion can be found in explorations 5.2, 5.3 and 5.4, and table 5.1 provides examples of yin and yang moments in Western dance.)

REVISITING COMPLEX MOVEMENT – THE DYNAMIC BALANCE OF PIROUETTE

The pirouette is a complex action requiring balance, strength, speed, rhythm and precision, and at the same time, successful turning requires additionally that we listen to the body. It can be challenging to find the balance between the ideal amount of control necessary and to listen in the moment and allow the body to autoadjust and surf the flow of the turn. The elusiveness of that dynamic balance provokes the most angst for dancers, concluded the study of the attentional focus of professional dancers (Guss-West and Wulf 2016). Successful turning is not so much a question of working more on control and technique as it is turning our attention to the role of the mind and the psychology of pirouettes. A clear attention and focus strategy is essential and can have the surprising effect of dissolving long-held mental blocks, alleviating pirouette angst and promoting easy, successful performance outcomes.

Letting go of our temptation to consciously control the verticality and learning to clear the mind of extraneous self-dialogue and critique, as in the Eastern no-mind principle, is perhaps the most essential skill for enhancing pirouette performance. Here we look at a couple of attention and breath strategies to enhance the adaptive balance and the potential speed of the turn and to minimize interfering pirouette stress.

The most challenging moment of the pirouette is the shift of weight, the transition from the preparatory phase to establish verticality within the first turn (Hopper et al. 2018). It's a dynamic transition that requires us to guide the attention clearly onto the intended movement outcome (i.e., the desired verticality or the clear rhythm of the multiple pirouettes we envisage [EF]). This allows the body's automatic, fast, reflexive control processes to function and adapt and make constant in-the-moment microadjustments to verticality and balance (figure 4.14). This transition can be mastered by listening to the body, through a process of implicit learning promoted by the use of simple EF cues because '. . . the balance achieved by dancers through the turns is not static but continually adaptive and specific to the individual dancer and movement' (Hopper et al. 2018, 237). The adaptive strategies of our body are completely individual and based on *our* body type and *our* strength.

Whatever our chosen EF cue for the pirouette – whether it is to focus on the vertical line of a wall in the studio, to push the floor away, to feel the two-way pull, to imagine a vertical red line through the centre, to recall a mental rehearsal of the rhythm of the ideal multiple pirouette or to imagine that we are surfing on the energy fountain – once we achieve our reflexive verticality, we are often tempted to release the EF from our mind rather than to refresh and reinforce it. This shift or release of our attention provokes an immediate loss of stability and capacity to autoadjust because we inevitably allow our attention to go somewhere else. The function of the EF is to guide, filter and simplify the attentional challenges and enhance the movement objective. It's essential then to continually reset and sustain the EF right to the end of the movement to assure successful microadjustments through to the conclusion and closing of the pirouette.

PIROUETTE PSYCHOLOGY

If pirouettes provoke performance stress, it's even more tempting to want to interfere with this reflexive process by doing more ourselves. We might add a few self-control cues such as pull in the abdominals, press down the shoulders or hold the back to the chosen external focus just for good measure. When we begin to bring our attention to our attention, we may also realize there is an entire self-related inner dialogue running in our head during stressful moments. We may find there are worries about our ability that we project *before* we attempt something and self-criticism or regrets *afterwards*. These additional IF instructions and the inner dialogue or self-commentaries devastate our focus and power and dissipate our energy, sending it off in multiple directions, undermining our best efforts to master any movement.

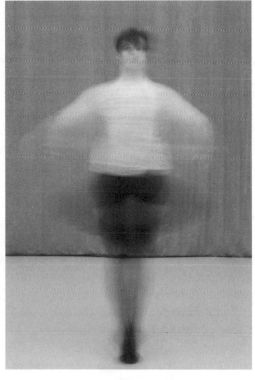

> We need to be aware that the mind is leading the Chi (energy) . . . not to push our form, for to do so will cause the body to be scattered and the movements uncoordinated. (Watts n.d., para 5)

This developing awareness and the process of clearing the mind of self-related thoughts of control

Figure 4.14   Surfing – microadjustments to verticality in a pirouette. (Ben)

or criticisms is one of the elements of high-performance sport psychology. Sometimes referred to as mindful practices or mindfulness, it permits the performer to be 100 per cent present in the moment, operating on full power, mind and body. This is the same desired state as that described in the Eastern movement mind state of no-mind. We need to develop the ability to identify and put to one side unhelpful thoughts, to clear the mind of extraneous dialogue and commentary, whether negative or positive, and at the same time learn to strengthen our attentional process. It's only human that unconscious or unhelpful thoughts pass through the mind, especially in movement, so it's important to begin to recognize *when* our thoughts are interrupting our movement and to develop strategies to reset our desired attentional EF control process and chosen focus or foci. (See chapter 5 for more on the no-mind state to promote maximum energy and for exercises to develop attention and clear the mind of disruptive thoughts.)

If you experience pirouette stress, then developing this no-mind state can have a significant impact on successful turning, particularly when the choreography demands multiple turns or a challenging extended series of turns. If nerves and stress cause an Olympic gymnast, for example, to mess up the first of a series of five challenging turns, they must have a strategy in place to empty the mind of all commentaries and reset their chosen attentional focus and bring 100 per cent attention to the present, to the remaining four turns. With such a strategy in hand, the gymnast can still potentially score 80 per cent for the series. When developing coping strategies with dance students for exam pirouette stress, they spontaneously called this approach goldfish brain. As the fish swims around the bowl, he has, anecdotally, no recall of having been there before on the previous turn, enabling him to attend afresh to his circumstances and surroundings. So, following an unsuccessful pirouette, the dancers would literally or metaphorically wipe their forehead and say 'goldfish brain', meaning forget it and move on. This goldfish brain image encapsulated the strategy and was successful for those vocational students. Perhaps you can think of another analogy for approaching each moment anew with a fresh mind and focus.

Another idea prevalent among dancers is the one-sided bias for turning. They might say something like, 'I've never been a good turner to the left'. The more we repeat this commentary to ourselves, the more embedded it becomes as a neural message, a kind of self-fulfilling prophecy that soon becomes our reality. There may, of course, be valid reasons for an imbalance. Many teachers still construct their class so that exercises *always* commence on the right and therefore the left falls as the second side or the other side, implying that it is somehow the secondary or inferior side. Many teachers also often ask dancers to repeat a skill, perhaps four times to the right and then often only once or

PIROUETTE – MAKING A THOUSAND, MILLION CORRECTIONS

Javier Torres, international teacher, choreographer, former professional dancer

For many years I hated doing pirouettes, especially en dehors. I think I got this panic from the perfection that my teacher wanted. I remember him saying 'you go up there, you just *hold* your position and if you lose it you fall straight like a tree'! And so, for a long time I could either do perfect pirouettes or none. But you know? When you go on stage you don't want to fall like a tree, so you're going to try to save the pirouette no matter what and for that you need to let your body react. If you're not taught that, you keep falling like a tree! It took me a long time to find another way because I kept training myself to 'hold like a tree'.

What helped me eventually was the connection to the breath. I had to forget my legs, the little toe, the knee, the passé and trust they would work. Then I managed to get up there with more of a sensation of freedom. Now I know that balance is not about striking the position, it's about making a thousand, million corrections constantly because your body keeps moving. David Howard, one of my most important teachers and a well-known personality of the dance world, would say 'finding the balance in a pirouette or in a static balance is like finding the right station on an old analogue radio: First you hear tzsh – zsh – zsh – sh and then suddenly a very clear voice says "And the good news of the day . . ."' I love this idea because it took away the static, and my body became alive whilst I was turning.

This is what dancers experience in tendu when we say 'sustain the spiral'. They are picturing that their body keeps moving whilst doing something seemingly still. I mean it's never still. If you allow your body to be alive – its wiser than you think – it will find the way to where we want it to be. This helped a lot. I would tell myself to 'allow' the pirouette, trust myself, breathe out and allow it.

twice to the left for lack of time. That alone represents a substantial 2-to-1 bias of right over left that will inevitably affect skills mastery.

Consider for a moment the training of a pianist: They play with two hands, left and right, and like dancers, they train each hand separately. The pianist, like the dancer, must eventually play one coherent piece of music with one body and one brain. Left and right integration needs to be seamless and without bias. A pianist can't suddenly say 'Oh sorry, I can't play that piece of music because my left hand is not as able as my right!' So too with dance. The separate sides need equal attention and respect in order to achieve the desired seamless integration and successful performance with our whole instrument.

Let's look at this with fresh eyes: I propose a completely different way of seeing this pirouette bias. Respect for the supporting or standing side is one of the foundations of Eastern movement that we have been discussing in dance practice. If you turn well to the right then it's thanks to the fact that your left leg provides stability and is excellent at supporting, and perhaps that's because it's had more practice. If you don't turn so well to the left, likewise, this is because your right leg is less proficient at providing stability. The right side simply doesn't get enough practice at supporting. Looked at this way, you can give thanks to the left for its excellent support, and then focus on developing the same respect and attention to support from the right for your pirouettes to the 'other' side.

In general, practicing a kind of daily 'amnesia' enhances integration quite rapidly. Rather than always reinforcing this polarity of good side versus bad side in any aspect of training, aim to 'zone out' and forget which side is practicing or mix them up a bit. Change your orientation in class or on the barre until you are confused about whether its left or right, good or bad, and focus only on the whole movement intention. To put the consequence of your daily choices into perspective, here's an experiment I conducted on myself. After dancing 40 years with a right bias, I chose to impose a left bias while training, so I always started first to the left. Within one month, the two sides were functioning equally, and within two months of proactive left training, the left became the dominant side. Changing habitual patterns of movement and well-established neural pathways can be accomplished at any age or skill level and is a matter of developing consciousness, making a choice and guiding attention.

PIROUETTE – POTENTIAL, POWER AND SPEED

We have brought our attention and energy to focus in the moment to develop the no-mind state and enhanced our adaptive verticality and fluidity by introducing a clear EF cue for ourselves. Now we can turn our attention to power and speed.

Two foundational EF elements from Eastern movement practice can have a significant impact on the explosive power of the pirouette: The coordination of the breath for optimum force production and the harnessing of natural resistance provided by jin energy. In chapter 3, we experienced the power, speed and constant sustain of the out-breath, which we can coordinate for movements that require these qualities. The power out-breath is the most adapted to facilitate the dynamic transition and initial turn phase of the pirouette when we want a speedy verticality. This initiating out-breath can support and sustain the pirouette throughout multiple rotations.

This means that the preparatory phase of the pirouette is essentially a moment of gathering potential for the turn. As you take your preparatory position, explore expanding against the demi-plié action and allow breath (and therefore energy) in to fill the energy highway and the body's cavities (see figure 4.15). This feeling of expanding against the demi-plié is sometimes referred to in dance as resisting the preparation or *not* sitting. The reason for the sensation of resisting is because the quality natural to jin energy (energy directed by the mind and our clear intention) is that of providing resistance. As we draw energy in and fill the lower energy centre, the substantial energy provides a buoyant resistance. In Eastern movement practice we suggest that gathering substantial jin energy in the lower body produces a resistance similar to pressing a large beach ball into water.

> While the pressure of pushing the ball is maintained, a resistance is felt, and when we release that pressure, the ball is repelled back out of the water. From the martial aspect, this jin absorbs the opponent's attack and then bounces him away. (Watts n.d.)

Looked out from the perspective of pirouettes, we expand, push and resist the substantial incoming energy and breath in preparation. As we push down and release that pressure with the power out-breath, we are repelled from the ground and explode into our verticality. Suspend any disbelief and approach your pirouettes with fresh eyes, open to new experiences and outcomes. As you first explore these foci and reverse breathing in your turning, you might be taken by surprise at the natural power and speed of the initiation. You have to be ready with your clear EF in mind to promote the verticality of the turns and to surf with the movement. Enjoy!

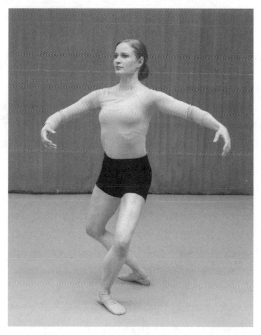

Figure 4.15   Gathering potential in the preparatory phase of a pirouette with the in-breath. (Emmi)

REVISITING COMPLEX MOVEMENT – THE EXPLOSIVE POWER OF ALLEGRO

Dazzling lower-limb movement and jumps at increasing heights require high power-out yang energy with quick-firing, autonomous, efficient muscles and often leave little time for yin energy and recuperation. Successful jumps require not only optimal force production, but dance also demands a sense of effort-lessness and buoyancy (ballon), precise form and expressive phrasing. When the movement phrase requires speed as well as power, a common response is to contract, to use *more* effort, hold the breath and increase tension in the joints. This more-is-more response triggers inappropriate muscular engagement and constricts and restrains energy flow inside, as we experienced in exploration 3.1. Far from producing more power and speed, this response produces slow, inconsistent movement that is quickly exhausted. A focus on fluidity, energy flow, space, breathing joints, coordinated breathing and minimum tension is essential for achieving the speed, agility and power demanded by allegro or lively, explosive dance phrases. 'Move with a clarity. Don't use force as a subject;' says international choreographer William Forsythe, 'force is not a subject. Speed and accuracy are a subject, but speed and accuracy without force' (National Ballet of Canada 2019).

Adopting a systematic external attentional focus strategy for allegro enables us to take advantage of precisely those benefits of maximum force production, fluidity, precision, speed and stamina. The dancers in the study of profes-sional dancer's attentional focus (Guss-West and Wulf 2016) demonstrated the greatest, spontaneous use of an EF in the ballistic jump, a grand jeté en avant. Explore lively jumps and allegro with any of the range of potential EF from figure 2.3 of your choice, from more tangible 'focus on the distance or the space created between the shapes and extensions' to a sensory EF or metaphoric imagery such as 'guide energy powerfully out through the extensions', 'jump over a lake' or 'take off with the back thrust of a rocket' (Guss-West and Wulf 2016). Effective EF cues or images should be clear and brief, encapsulating essential information about the movement objective: the form, the quality or the dynamics that can be easily sustained whilst dancing.

Elements from Eastern movement practice can further enhance the effort-lessness, power, precision of the form, and artistry of allegro movement. In addition to the use of an EF, you can use any of the several other Eastern movement attentional foci we have explored:

- Respect the whole to promote compelling, cohesive movement and power.
- Expand into speed and maintain breathing joints to promote fluidity and agility.
- Coordinate the breath to promote power, precision and musicality.

- Harness the natural resistance of jin energy and reverse breathing as used in the pirouette preparation for an explosive take-off.
- Seek yin recuperation in motion for increased stamina.

SPEED AND PRECISION – SMALL JUMPS OR PETIT ALLEGRO AND BEATS

Fast, precise lower-limb agility is first developed at the barre in classical Western dance training. These foundational actions embed our habitual approach to speed and precision.

Despite or precisely because of the desire for lightning-fast speed, we need to respect and maintain energy in the whole system and not fragment our attention, however tempting that may be to send energy only downwards into the demanding lower-limb actions. Allow the lower energy centre to circulate energy through the whole energy system (the energy highway, heart and crown centres, and beyond) throughout extended phrases. This promotes a cohesive, fast, fluid movement with minimum tension.

To enhance fast, accented or beaten actions such as a glissé (slide), piqué (stab), frappé (strike) or brisé (broken), take the moment of extension as a yang, power-out movement, coordinated with the outgoing breath. Focusing on each thorough out-breath during moments of speed and precision will facilitate the expansion of the in-breath as a reflex action, assuring optimal oxygenation, energy and stamina. As choreographic phrases become more complex with multiple glissés, fast frappés or battement actions, we need to attend to whole musical phrases and the flow and continuity of the multiple movements rather than a series of individual parts. Imagine playing a flute or trumpet, singing or even swimming the crawl. The breath is coordinated with the movement based on the demands of the action. One long, sustained out-breath can carry through multiple musical bars or, in the case of dance, lower-limb actions. If glissés or petit allegro beats, such as brisés, are arranged in rapid groups of threes or petit battement in a continuum of sevens or more, choosing to coordinate that with one sustained out-breath throughout the long, multiple-movement phrase promotes the stability, support, length, quality, continuity, speed, fluidity and musicality of the action.

EXPLOSIVE POWER – MEDIUM JUMPS OR MEDIUM ALLEGRO

In short fast jumps such as sautés, in beaten jumps and in extensive medium allegro phrases, consciously using the natural resistance of jin energy and reverse breathing enhances a fast, explosive action with minimum effort.

EXPLORATION 4.8 – EXPLOSIVE POWER

Let's experiment with a series of simple sautés in first position. So that we have a good base for comparison, take one or two series of six or eight jumps in first as you would do normally without thinking. Take a moment to notice how that felt: breathing, height, heaviness or lightness, stamina.

Let's take that again and this time apply some of the Eastern movement practice concepts we've looked at here and in chapter 3. Respecting the whole, start by circulating energy throughout the whole system, either using a preparatory breathing port de bras to gather energy (figure 4.3) or the large circulation of energy (figure 4.1).

Expand, make space and allow energy and breath in as you sink down and demi-plié. Sense the counterrise of the substantial energy in the lower energy centre like a beach ball rising in the water. Sense a resistance as you maintain the ball in the water. With the power out-breath, push down against the ball of energy into the water in one coordinated action and send it down and far away from you. Explosive jin power repels you from the ground. The out-breath continues throughout the elevation, feeling propelled like a rocket. Expand, allow breath in as you descend to land, demi-plié, resist the rising energy or ball in the water and push down and out to jump again.

Test a continuous, rhythmic series of six or eight sautés with this coordination of the breath and the energy, and then relax. What did you notice this time? Are you out of breath? How did it feel in terms of effort? Did you notice a change in jump height? In landing quality? In your stamina? Could you have kept going longer? Did you observe anything else? Perhaps take the series once again and then take a moment to jot down immediate thoughts and any differences from your first, habitual approach.

This reverse breathing logic can be applied to any small to medium jump for an explosive quality (see figure 4.16). The out-breath pushing energy down into the earth like a rocket's back thrust coordinates with the extension of the movement in assemblé, brisé or coupé fouetté raccourci, for example. Using this reverse power-out, yang breathing to achieve optimal explosive power in the jump brings many additional benefits. It means that the following reflexive incoming breath is also coordinated supporting the continuity of the technique and desired qualities. The incoming breath acts as a natural support for the joints and spine, cushioning the landings and assuring the quality of ballon or buoyancy. Coordinated in this way, the in-breath replenishes energy and at the same time provides the preparatory resistance necessary for the following jump.

Eastern movement practice reminds us to experiment and to be flexible with the use of the breath. The coordinated breath simply acts as a pump to facilitate the flow of energy through the body and beyond. The take-off moment of a glissade or sissonne, for example, if coordinated with the out-breath in this reverse breathing is fast, darting and dynamic; whereas, when the take-off is coordinated with the in-breath, they are not as explosive or high but have another softer, more lyrical quality. As you experiment, coordinate the breath to support optimal energy flow *and* the desired artistic outcome. The coordination of the breath with the demands of the movement objective naturally becomes more fluent with practice; however, you will experience immediate, palpable differences in jump facility as you begin to explore and implement reverse breathing preparation and push off.

BALLISTIC POWER – BIG JUMPS OR GRAND ALLEGRO

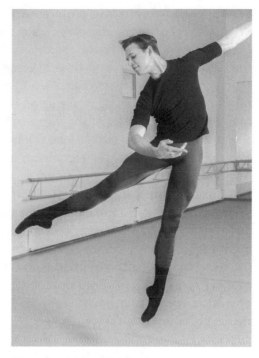

Figure 4.16   Explosive power – repelled from the ground with jin energy. (Ben)

Grand allegro, or big jumps, are often thought of as the culmination of a dancer's technical prowess. They require not only complete physical mastery but also appropriate mental and attentional focus preparation.

> Jumps should show the line of the position in the air. . . . They may be taken in all directions and alignments, and in straight lines, curves or circles. (Ryman 2008, 79)

Given the dimensional complexity of big jumps, the attention to the whole movement trajectory in space and its mental rehearsal are key to taking jump performance to the next level. A clear EF provides a blueprint for the body to follow, allowing for automatic, optimum muscular engagement and fast reflexive adaptive movements. If you do not already use it, you might introduce mental rehearsal as a chosen EF type (see figure 2.3). For example, re-create and imagine the whole form in space: the directions, the flow, the connections, the breathing and the optimal pathway of the jump in preparation. Tracing 'in our "mind's-eye" the gyroscopic relationship of arcs, curves and lines of energy as we project them out in space' (Guss-West 2014, 134) provides a blueprint or road map that enables the ideal precise, cohesive, three-dimensional aerial form and trajectory when in motion. Successful grand allegro also requires an immense musicality and embodiment of rhythm. For many dancers, a simple EF focus on the musicality of the preparation and the energy of the music in the jump is sufficient to guide the desired dynamics and flow of energy.

Reverse breathing as we explored for medium jumps harnesses the resistance of jin energy in the preparation for the explosive power-out in the initial take-off phase. Several of the dancers interviewed for the book suggest that this preparatory in-breath is already built into Western classical ballet in the allongé (elongation) – the expansion and lengthening in preparation for the big jump, which is an integral part of grand allegro.

Continue the yang power out-breath to the height of the elevation. When you sense you are close to the turning point of the body mass in the air, expand and allow breath and energy in against the pull of gravity. The incoming jin energy and oxygen sustain that glorious suspended moment in the air that is so often alluded to by the accompanying rallentando in the music (figure 4.17). As you descend, depending on the speed of the series of jumps you can either sustain the expansion and in-breath to support the landing and provide the resistance directly for the next power-out elevation, or you can manage musical breaths: out (descending), a drawn out in-breath (landing and preparation) and out (take-off). In a long, demanding series of big jumps, this additional attention to reverse breathing ensures replenishment of energy, increasing stamina and promotion of enhanced movement quality and flow. Phrases take on another dimension; rather than being the simple sum of the individual parts (Martin 2019), they become one whole fluid, expressive statement directing, sculpting and playing with the universal qualities of energy and air.

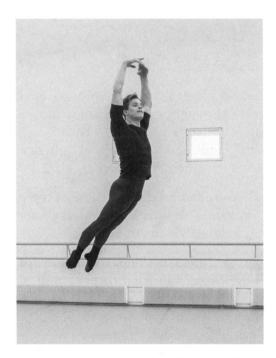

Figure 4.17   Coordinating breathing for maximum power, energy recuperation and musicality. (Ben)

REFLECTION PROMPTS

Were you able to suspend your disbeliefs during this chapter and approach the familiar with fresh eyes? This chapter offered lots of different perspectives to consider. Which concepts or images particularly spoke to you? Take a look back through your notes as you experimented with the concepts and explorations in this chapter: surfing on the energy fountain to dynamically balance (exploration 4.3), leading with the mind to unfold the extended leg – developpé (exploration 4.4), sensing the five simultaneous directions of the arabesque (exploration 4.5), using the no-mind state in pirouette, coordinating the gather and give cycle of adage (exploration 4.7) or using reverse breathing for explosive power (exploration 4.8).

Jot down new or creative thoughts that surfaced as you experimented. Did you have an aha! moment that revealed how you habitually approach particular movements or how you'd like to approach particular movements? Awareness is half of the journey to successful implementation, so be patient with yourself. At first, simply become aware of when your habitual way of approaching takes over. See if you can reset the mind and guide the attention, energy and breath to support your chosen approach.

The familiar foundations and movements we revisited in this chapter are just a few examples. The EF and Eastern movement concepts can be applied logically to any dance demands, from initial learning of the fundamentals to mastering and refining artistic details. How might you apply some of the concepts to the following?

- A plié exercise. How might you use the gather-and-give energy cycle throughout the exercise? Which energy centres do you connect with?

- A grand battement exercise. Which is the yang moment of the movement? If grand battement is a preparation for big jumps, how would you apply the logic of the breathing? What would be an optimum coordination of the out and the in? Why?

- A fondu exercise. Choose one or two EF types – real, tangible, sensory or imaginary – that would support the desired movement outcomes, qualities or form of the exercise.

Take from the elements that attract you today and leave the rest. Begin to experiment with them in your dancing and teaching. Once they become more fluent, dip back into this chapter and see whether other concepts resonate with you at that time. Remember: 'If you always do what you always did, you will always get what you always got' (Quote Investigator n.d.). So there are only positives that can come from deciding to open and give a little time and space of attention to new ways of seeing and we find that 'there art, there beauty is' (Watson 2017, 142).

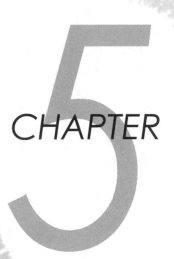

5
CHAPTER

REFOCUS MIND, REPLENISH ENERGY

If you begin to be aware, you begin to feel a new energy in you, a new fire, a new life. And because of this new life, new power, new energy, many things which were dominating you just dissolve.

Osho (n.d.)

*I*n chapter 3 we explored the foundations of an Eastern approach and the synergetic roles of attention, focus, energy and breath in movement. We touched on universal laws of movement and explored that all movement is in fact made up of just two possible actions or contrasting states that are described as either yin or yang. Yin is a moment of expanding, of making space and allowing 'potential' (oxygen and energy) to flow into our organism. Yang is a moment of contracting to provoke explosive or sustained outward power, like the firing of an engine. A multitude of binary movements activate our heart, our muscles, our lungs and our brain, expanding and contracting to pump oxygen, nutrients and energy through our thoughts, our movements and beyond. By respecting both the yang and the yin moments and attending to their contrasting qualities, we promote an optimum, constant flow of energy and sustained power throughout our organism.

You have probably already considered recovery activities for *after* physical dance exertion; however, it would be wise to take a look at energy management *in* motion itself. Finding the balance between yang and yin *whilst* dancing assures your energy reserves, your stamina and long-term staying power in the moment. This balancing of energy in motion is possible and natural in dance because of its human artistic components: the relationship to musicians, to music, to rhythm, to expression and to breath. The structure of dance phrasing is grounded in our humanness, on the yin and yang of artistic expression. Dance is not a race. The fastest dancer that finishes the work ahead of the others is not considered the most successful as they would be in sport, but instead would be considered the one who can't keep to the desired phrasing and musical timing! We have a wonderful opportunity to breathe new life and new energy into the humanness of our dance to enhance both our physical performance and also to develop our expression and our communication through our instrument and its movements.

In this chapter we look at foundational attention, focus, energy and breath techniques for energy management that you might like to try to sustain and replenish energy whilst dancing. We also begin to explore the process of attention in action and review our current attention skills and our ability to quiet and reset the mind, displacing depleting self-talk and disruptive thoughts whilst dancing. Lastly, we look at how to close down the dancing body for the day when we are done in order to conserve vital energy. Given the predominantly yang demands of Western dance styles and training and the relatively limited attention to the yin moments of recuperation and replenishing energy in action, the Western dancer can be prone to energy depletion, exhaustion and, if left unaddressed, eventually to chronic fatigue or burnout.

In preparation, like when moving the stone (exploration 3.1), first let's consider your typical energy expenditure and review your current sense of appropriate effort in any movement. As you might do in your own home to manage your spending and consumption, you want to become conscious of just how much energy you are using or potentially wasting and become smarter and more economical. If you have 'all the lights on in your house' all of the time, then you are not being economic nor moving as effectively as you are capable of. Muscular engagement is expensive, and contracted or held muscles block the efficient flow of energy in the body. Successful movement and energy management means finding the balance between minimum muscular engagement and contraction, expansion and release. You might start by introducing the practice of scanning for tension before you start to dance.

EXPLORATION 5.1 – PREPARATORY SCAN

This circular scan takes just a few seconds as you stand in preparation. Take your attention to the sensations in your body and ask yourself are all these *lights that are on* – muscles that are engaged – really necessary for this task? Consciously *switch off* one or two. Check for superficial holding, one area after another, in a circular sweep. Scan the shoulders, the occipital area, the face, the throat, the chest, the diaphragm, the wrists, the thumbs, the thighs, the ankles, the toes, the outer gluteus muscles and across the sacrum. Continue your circular scan back up through the spine to the occipital bone. Simply allow unnecessary holding to release until you arrive at a sense of what feels like the minimum essential that is appropriate for the task. As you introduce this into your daily practice, focus on the circular flow of the scan and the sensation of tension or holding, then the release and expansion to maintain your external attentional focus.

You can do this as often as you need in class or rehearsal until your body begins to reset its learnt perception of appropriate effort. This circular scan becomes a natural part of dance readiness and can take a matter of seconds once you become aware of your habitual holding patterns. In classical ballet, for instance, it could be effectively done with the preparatory breathing port de bras at the beginning of an exercise or variation. Now that your energy can flow, let's move on to replenishing energy in motion.

REPLENISHING ENERGY IN DANCE

Developing awareness is already half of the journey towards effective energy management. At first simply start by acknowledging and reaffirming to yourself daily that to dance with optimum power and stamina, it's just as important to let go, release, expand and allow space in the body as it is to contract and push outwards. Begin to play with the two synergistic states of yin and yang. Become aware of and identify them in a dance phrase. Is it possible to give them both equal attention? There are no hard and fast rules with energy. Which movements are potentially yin and which are definitely yang will vary based on the intention of the movement and the desired movement quality as much as it will be based on your personal choice and expression. As a simple guide, however, consider that most highlights, the so-called photo moments, in dance tend to be yang. The natural yin movements, or neutral moments as I refer to them, typically don't require high energy, there is no action highlight or precise extended line to achieve. There's no sustained balance or explosive jump. Yin moments are transition, supporting or preparatory moments of dance – the journey between two yang highpoints. Neutral, or yin, movements are foundational to the flow and structure of a dance phrase and are always present once we start to focus on them. The yang and yin moments typically alternate in a continuum of energy renewal. As you first experiment, the most accessible yin moments you will find are in a breathing port de bras preparation, in the preparatory demi-plié, the adage fondu moment or temps liés connecting movements. These are all excellent moments in which we potentially have a little more time to bring our attention to the sensation of a breathing expansion. As your ability to manage energy renewal in the yin movements becomes more fluent, however, even the most fleeting of glissades or briefest coupé transfer of weight become a snatched opportunity to expand and refresh energy. See table 5.1 for examples of potential yang and yin moments in Western dance.

TABLE 5.1   Potential Yang and Yin Moments in Western Dance

YANG: ACTION, POWER, OUT-BREATH	YIN: ALLOWING, REPLENISHING, IN-BREATH
Giving, extending lines of energy out from a port de bras	Gathering, lifting, transitioning energy in a port de bras
A sustained contraction and reach	A sustained elongation and unrolling or circling out of a grand port de bras to support the spine
Unfolding the leg (developpé) into a precise, high line	The fondu moment, returning to the centre support or the rotation transition in adage, replenishing in preparation for the next extension out
The push down to rise in balance	The supported lowering to the floor (through the foot) of temps liés or sustained transfer of weight and demi-plié preparation
The upward throw of the grand battement action	The supported lowering action of the leg from grand battement or arabesque
The push off into pirouette	The demi-plié and preparation for pirouette
The push off into a big jump	The preparatory demi-plié, glissade or allongé before a big jump
Relevé and echappé actions, dynamic rises	Coupé or quick change of weight

Some dance styles encourage carrying the weight far forward over the forefoot so the dancer is constantly ready for action. In Eastern practice, shifting the weight forwards and engaging the musculature for action, on quarter or demi-pointe, pumps higher-power yang energy through the system (Chuen 2003). If used continuously, this stance will deplete the system of energy. If you regularly use this weight-forward, active stance or have high demands for demi-pointe, be sure to find a conscious moment from time to time to connect with the floor and the earth with the weight on the whole foot (yin) as a contrast. Connect an instant with the pressure of the floor as the movement closes or whenever possible to maintain the replenishing yin–yang continuum.

As you begin to focus on expanding and allowing breath and energy in during the transitional, supporting and preparatory yin moments in dance, you will not only encounter consistent energy and improved stamina, but you will also find that this attention promotes enhanced balance, fluidity and support throughout these connecting movements. The expansion and the in-breath provide support for a fluid transition, creating space in the spine and cushioning a lowering that further enhances the quality of the overall performance.

REPLENISHING TECHNIQUES

During movement, energy can be consistently drawn from the surrounding universal energy field and circulated through our movements and beyond using the breath, the attention and the mind. Initially, simply focusing on the coordination of the breathing cycle (explorations 3.4, 3.5, 4.1 and 4.7) will immediately increase energy flow through your movement. The more consistently and thoroughly you use the out-breath for the power-out moments to fuel the vital organs and the extremities, the greater will be the capacity of the reflexive action of the in-breath to replenish potential: oxygen, energy and nutrients.

To replenish energy *whilst* dancing, take a look at explorations 5.2, 5.3 and 5.4, which provide simple techniques you can practice to ensure constant energy and improved stamina. Try the replenishing techniques first from a still, standing position to focus more easily on the movement of the attention, the breath and the sensations of energy flow. In these still versions, aim to identify clear, proprioceptive sensations that you will be able to recall and apply later in dance practice.

First create and store your own limitless source of energy in the lower-body energy centre: dan tien, or bras bas, area (exploration 5.2). The concept of cultivating your own source of energy in the lower energy centre is fundamental to Eastern movement practice. The continuous replenishing of energy in the body is a daily practice. Learning lower energy centre or belly breathing will establish your own inner energy store that you can top up with energy from the universal field with every breath you take. It's your own personal, constant source that fills your being and sustains the demands of your actions.

The more that you can attend to the sensations you experience in the explorations and the more key words or images you can capture to describe and cue them for yourself, the quicker you will be able to recall and implement them *whilst* in motion in class or in rehearsal amidst so many other stimuli vying for your attention. You might find you need to repeat the exploration a couple of times before you feel that the proprioceptive sensations are registered clearly in your body.

EXPLORATION 5.2 – THE CONSTANT ENERGY SOURCE – LOWER ENERGY–CENTRE BREATHING

Find a quiet space where you will not be interrupted. Standing in an open parallel or a natural first position, whichever is more comfortable, place one palm firmly on your belly under your tummy button and place the other lightly on top on the back of the first hand as if you wanted to contain all the energy that is in your lower body. Allow space around the body for air and energy to circulate and space between the vertebrae through the spine. The head lightly balanced on the top. Slowly sink into a demi-plié, and breathe. Can you feel the heat from your hands? Take your attention and your breathing down to where you can feel the heat. Breathe for a moment, feeling the heat, and notice that as you allow breath in, the belly expands and rises a little, moving your hands. As you breathe out, press a little to encourage complete emptying. Breathe for a moment with the heat and the motion of the rise and the press. Did the heat increase? Where you feel the warmth, imagine a bright, revolving sunlight energy that is golden yellow, warm orange or brilliant white. It is a dancing inner sunlight that fills your lower body, turning and moving. It is bright and warm under your hands.

Allow the sunlight energy to fill your lower body, revolving and making space. Allow it through the sacrum and the lower spine and through the skin, circling around you. With each in-breath, top up the revolving, sunlight energy. With each out-breath, send it gently through your body. Peel the hands gradually away from the belly just a couple of centimetres to allow space. Encircle the growing, dancing energy moving gradually further away with each in-breath until your hands slowly separate. Your arms are full of bright sunlight energy, revolving and dancing around, behind and through your body. Embrace it, and breathe a moment with all the sensations.

Releasing, turn your palms slowly, opening them out to allow excessive heat and energy to return to the universal energy field. With an out-breath, push into the floor and straighten. Shake out, jump about, stretch or whatever you need to do to get all that renewed energy into your system.

That was a long concentration! Well done. Take a moment before you go on to jot down immediate impressions and sensations – a few key words to take with you back into dance practice. What was a vivid sensation for you? The heat? The feeling of expansion? The revolving? The calm rhythm? The vibrant colours? Choose two or three key words you can use to access and recapture the sensations quickly in another environment.

If you found yourself yawning as you practiced this preparatory energy exploration, there's no need to suppress or to fight the yawn. It's a normal reaction to increased energy and oxygen flow and is the body's quickest way to release stuck energy, toxins and carbon dioxide. So yawn thoroughly and enjoy! Remember to drink plenty of water after energy exploration to help the system process toxins that have shifted. Expect the unexpected. Renewed energy will flow where it is most needed, so if you were feeling sluggish and slow, for example, you might find yourself suddenly motivated for action, and if you were feeling hyperactive or stressed, you might find yourself calmer or even sleepy and in need of restorative sleep. Listen to your body and try to profit from the healing aspects of this practice.

Replenishing energy in motion can eventually be realized independently of the breathing cycle, like the concept of breathing joints. In fact, as with the ports de bras in chapter 4, chi kung practice suggests that for mobilizing energy, it's important to avoid getting too dependent on a fixed breathing pattern (Brecher 2001). The renewal of energy can be consciously realized with the mind and the attention alone. *Where the mind will go, blood and energy follow* (Quian 2017). Energy can easily flow through the 99.9 per cent space that makes up our cells, passing without resistance through the largest organ, the skin's porous surface. Whilst in motion, energy renewal can be effectively activated by taking the attention to a couple of key energy gateways in the body.

Central to energy renewal in motion is the spine, which quite simply *is* our 'energy highway'. The spine houses all of our central nervous system and electrical circuitry, running information at the speed of light to and fro between the brain and the extremities. The typical dance and chi kung posture of elongated spine with space between the vertebrae is ideal for facilitating maximum energy flow.

Having created a personal store of lower-body energy in exploration 5.2, let's move on to explore how to circulate that energy effectively through the energy highway and the vital organs with a practice called the small circulation of energy. Similar to the large circulation of energy (figure 4.1) for the effortless two-way pull of our postural alignment, this simple, mind-led technique keeps energy circulating through all the sensory and vital organs whilst you are dancing. It can easily be combined with the preparatory circular scan for tension described in exploration 5.1. It can be coordinated anywhere with any in- and out-breath cycle: whilst walking down the road, waiting in a queue or lying in bed or during any appropriate moment in a dance phrase to maintain optimum power.

EXPLORATION 5.3 – THE SMALL CIRCULATION OF ENERGY

Take an open parallel or a natural first position again, arms loosely by your sides or hands arranged on the belly as in exploration 5.2. Take a moment to make space

(continued)

EXPLORATION 5.3 (continued)

and allow air and energy to circulate around the body and take your breathing down into the lower-body energy centre. When you are ready, breathe out, and lead energy from your lower energy centre forwards and down to circle around the torso. As you expand and allow breath in, send the energy upwards through the spine and through the back of the head like a powerful water fountain that lifts and floats the vertebrae. With the out-breath, imagine the water of the fountain cascading down, stroking across your face, dropping around your shoulders and softening the chest and the diaphragm. (See figure 5.1.) Let it flow downwards to circle the torso again, enlivening and lengthening the spine with the next expansion and influx of breath in a continuous circling motion (Prath 2019; Lee 2016).

This circulation is an effective tool for promoting the seemingly contradictory demands of dance: to be powerful and yet fluidly expressive in the same movement. The upward lift of the in-breath assures support for action. The cascading, waterlike energy of the out-breath softens the front of the body, the face and the chest, dissolving tension to allow the transmission of emotions and artistic expression.

Later, you might try the small circulation of energy with reverse breathing. You can send a powerful out-breath and energy up through the back of the body, shooting through the spine like a geyser out of the earth, lifting the vertebrae and bringing dynamic energy and space. The spine is strong and yet fluid with the fish-like qualities. With the expansion and in-breath, imagine that water cascades down across the face and chest as before, but this time supporting and yet softening at the same time. As the wave of the in-breath completes, circle energy around the torso and prepare to power-out up through the spine and beyond and so on. If you experiment with both breathing coordinations in the cycle, you may notice that reverse breathing produces a different quality energy and effect and a sense of readiness for high yang action. Both will replenish and activate energy in your system as you dance, so explore and use whichever seems most appropriate for the demands of the movement that you are preparing.

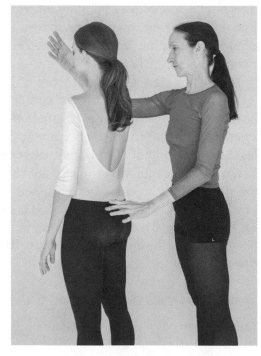

Figure 5.1   The small circulation of energy. (Kailey and Clare)

As in Eastern movement practice, the Western classical dance posture focuses attention beyond the spine to the two bony plates at the top and bottom of the energy highway: the occipital area and the sacrum. Classical posture requires a lengthening or opening of the sacrum area, often referred to as a balanced or neutral pelvis (Ryman 2008) and an elongation and lifting of the occipital area where it joins the spine. These two bony plates are key energy access points in Eastern movement practice, serving and replenishing the flow of energy through the spine whilst in motion. To facilitate this renewal, the sacrum and the occipital area would ideally be fluid joints that are open and breathing.

The sacrum is situated in the back of our lower energy centre and at one time was considered sacred, hence its name the 'sacred bone', because it protects all the vital organs necessary for the creation of life (MedicineNet n.d.). It is essential that this area can open and breathe whilst moving, particularly during movement phrases of sustained effort, in order to ensure the renewal of energy to the lower energy store and through the vital organs and lower limbs. The lightly lifted occipital bone effectively permits the bony area and its joints to open and breathe and absorb energy, serving and replenishing energy flow to the brain and vital sensory organs. These two areas are typically contracted and closed off when applying inappropriate effort or a muscle-led approach to a movement task. This limits the renewal of energy through the whole system, and the system becomes weakened and depleted of energy or exhausted.

In the following explorations we take our attention to the sacrum and occipital areas to develop the proprioceptive sensations of opening and breathing through the joints. The difference between closed off and open in physical terms may be less than a couple of millimetres. So we bring our attention not to the physical action but to the direction of our intention and the sensation of allowing energy to flow through these open access points to boost and replenish the energy supply through the spine, the brain, the nervous system and the sensitive upper-body vital organs.

We are often unaware of just how much holding and tension the sacrum is carrying from our efforts. Taking our attention to the sacrum is perhaps the easiest place to start to immediately capture the contrasting sensation of opening and allowing the area to expand. I imagine the energy highway like the strings of a cello, with sound and energy resounding and flowing the length of the spine and beyond. The lower touch of the strings (sacrum) gives a deeper bass-sounding energy, with stronger, more readily detectable vibrations; whereas the higher touch (occipital bone) has a lighter, more ethereal sound and vibration that can be more subtle to sense at first. To explore sacrum breathing, you need a willing partner dancer to experiment with you. If you are a teacher, this is a wonderful mindful class exercise to be taken in pairs.

EXPLORATION 5.4 – SACRUM AND OCCIPITAL BREATHING

In this two-part exploration we will be working with the hands, the touch and the warmth of a partner dancer to provide a perfect external focus, allowing us to sensitize and breathe through the joints and the surface of the sacrum and the occipital areas. The EF of touch can be recalled later and will be easily accessible to you at any moment in your dancing. You will be able to recapture the hologram of sensations: the pressure and warmth of their hands, the proprioceptive sense of expansion, opening and breathing and the appropriate tension and effort in your own posture. An exploration may take 10 minutes for each dancer and yet will provide a lasting resource to support you through a life-long career of healthful dancing. Both dancers will get to play each role: that of the receiving, sensing partner and that of the active, doing partner.

5.4(a) – Sacrum Breathing

With your partner, decide who will be the receiving partner first and who will be the active partner who provides the external, proprioceptive attentional focus.

If you are the receiving partner, stand in open parallel with your arms hanging loosely by your sides. Allow space for air to flow around the body and space between the vertebrae through the spine. With the head lightly balancing on the top, slowly sink to a demi-plié. Lower your gaze or close your eyes and breathe.

If you are the active partner, make a butterfly with your hands (see figure 5.2), touching the heel of the hands together. Place the hands firmly on the sacrum of your partner, giving a slight pressure downwards rather than inwards. Get comfortable in this position by taking a secure open stance in demi-plié, and allow your elbows and shoulders to be fluid and breathe easily and naturally so you don't transfer any tension from your body into your partner.

Receiving Dancer: Can you feel the pressure from the hands? Take your attention and your breathing down into the lower body to where you can feel the pressure. Can you feel the heat from the hands? Feel the heat expanding the area as you breathe, and imagine that you could

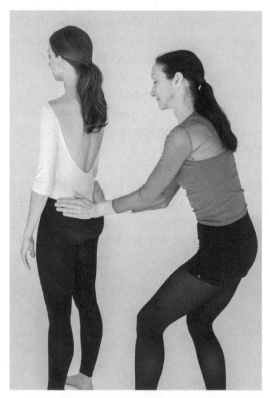

Figure 5.2   Receiving dancer and active dancer prepare the sacrum breathing exploration. (Kailey and Clare)

take the breath towards the heat. Allow the breath to pass through the bone and through the muscle and the skin into the palms of your partner. Breathe there for a moment together.

Active Dancer: You may notice an expansion under your hands and the heat increasing. After a moment spent with the breathing, begin to peel the hands away from the sacrum very gradually to about five centimetres (two inches) away from the surface of the skin. Pause and breathe for a moment.

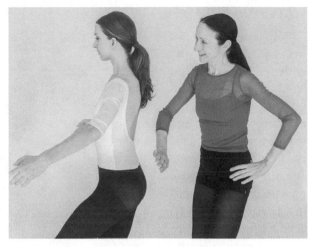

Figure 5.3   The active dancer moves gradually away to give space for sacrum breathing. (Kailey and Clare)

Receiving Dancer: What do you feel as the hands make space? Continue to breathe through the body, through the bones, through the muscles and beyond into the palms. Pause and breathe together a moment.

Active Dancer: Again, move away gradually to about 15 centimetres (6 inches) away from the body. Pause and breathe together a moment (see figure 5.3).

Receiving Dancer: Can you still feel the hands? The warmth?

Active Dancer: Gradually move your hands further and further away with each slow expansion and in-breath. Take a few steps away until you are far from your partner, and then relax.

Receiving Dancer: Staying focused on the warmth, continue breathing into the 'hands' you can still sense, expanding with each in-breath. When you are ready, come out of the exercise by stretching the extremities first and then the whole body. Open your eyes and come back into the room. Turn around and see just how far your partner is from you! You felt that they were right there with you, no? Thank your partner and exchange a few of the sensations and your observations.

Now switch roles and repeat the exploration. Take your time. Each one of us is different and takes a different amount of time to be able to focus on our sensations.

Afterwards be sure to jot down a few key words that came to mind or that you discussed with your partner to describe the sensations. This will help you embed the proprioceptive sensations and embody the learning from the new experience.

5.4(b) – Occipital Breathing

As you did for sacrum breathing, if you are the receiving partner, stand in open parallel with your arms hanging loosely by your sides. Allow space for air to flow around the body. This time remain standing straight without demi-plié if you prefer; however, keep the knees and joints soft and breathing.

(continued)

EXPLORATION 5.4 *(continued)*

The active dancer makes the butterfly with the hands to cup lightly around the occipital bone, behind the ears and under the hair if your partner has a ponytail or bun, giving the slightest pressure upwards rather than inwards (figure 5.4). Get comfortable in this position, breathe easily and naturally, and allow your hands to flow around the bone like water without transferring any tension.

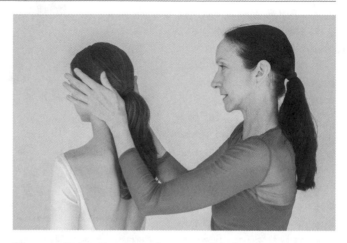

Figure 5.4   Receiving dancer and active dancer prepare the occipital breathing exploration. (Kailey and Clare)

Receiving Dancer: Can you feel the light pressure from the hands? Take your breathing and your attention to where you can feel the pressure. Can you feel heat? Imagine that you could take the breath towards the heat, and allow the breath to pass through the bone, through the muscle and through the skin into the palms of your partner. Breathe there for a moment together into the hands.

Active Dancer: Continue the same as for sacrum breathing, taking your time to gradually peel your hands slightly away from the bone while still cupping the area. Breathe there together for a moment, and then move a little further. Pause and then gradually move away with each expansion and in-breath.

Receiving Dancer: When you are ready, stretch the extremities and the spine and take a big yawn, whatever you need to bring yourself back into the room.

Thank your partner and exchange a few observations from the exploration, jotting down key words about the sensations whilst they are clear in your mind. Did you notice that the occipital bone gave sensations different from the sacrum? A different quality energy? Were the opening sensations lighter or more subtle to detect? Did images come to mind as you were breathing and exploring? If yes, be sure to jot them down because these will serve as effective EF to cue yourself later to open the occipital area whilst dancing.

As you first begin to experiment in your dance practice, you may have a sense that it's counterintuitive to allow these areas to expand and breathe as you address demanding movement phrases. Once you experience that there is no loss of power, however, rather a surge of sustained energy, as in the mind-led, less-is-more arm press (exploration 3.7), a greater sense of lightness and ease, and increased fluidity and range of motion, you will actively seek the moments in a phrase in which you can implement these new replenishing energy techniques.

You may wish to return to the still, standing explorations from time to time to refresh the imprint of the proprioceptive sensations of expansion or lightness and assist your recall of the sensation of circulating energy whilst dancing. The explorations can also be practiced at any time to replenish and store energy in the lower body or to induce an energized state of calm before a performance.

CONSERVING ENERGY IN DANCE

If we think about the structure of any Western dance class, it typically begins relatively gently and offers plenty of opportunity for breathing and balancing yin energy. Once we become warm or, in chi kung terms, once we move energy and blood higher through the body and charge it with our conscious breathing, it becomes more and more yang (heat, action, power). At this point, the intensity and the demands of the dance class increase. As a typical Western class progresses, we increasingly shift energy through our movements, opening energy centres, powering-out and sending energy in every imaginable direction.

Eastern movement practice instructs us that *what is lifted must be lowered* (Brecher 2001). Sustaining high energy around the heart (middle dan tien or first position) and the crown energy centre (upper dan tien, fifth position, or couronne area) increases pressure and heat around the delicate sensory organs and opens the crown to universal energy.

It's important, therefore, to be aware of constantly circulating energy. In chi kung practice, as in traditional classical ballet, all ports de bras are designed to lower and close in lower dan tien or bras bas, drawing excessive heat and energy away from the brain and the nervous system and lowering it where it may be safely stored at the end of each exercise. In Eastern practice, it is considered unwise to leave the upper body charged with yang energy because this leads to yin deficiency and provokes potential imbalances such as irritability, inability to focus or emotional instability. A habitually overcharged crown, brain and upper body would, according to Eastern medicine, result in problems of the more delicate upper-body organs: the heart, nervous system, emotions and brain. A fiery yang imbalance in the upper body eventually leads to physical and mental burnout. Eastern medicine identifies that one of the chronic issues of our Western society is that we are too highly charged with energy in the head and upper body through too much cognitive and sensory stimulation and that we practice insufficient physical movement and grounding of energy to restore our yin-to-yang balance.

Not all dance styles consciously address this need to bring excessive heat and energy downwards – literally to cool down – and close at the end of a demanding session. It's one of the traditional functions of the closing in chi kung and of the closing reverence in classical ballet. Using an inwards, en dedans port de bras, we bring energy downwards and draw heat and yang energy away from the brain, eyes and heart. We lower it through the body to store it in the lower energy centre, the bras bas area. (See figure 5.5.) Another function of a closing or reverence is to close down the principal energy centres of the crown, the heart and the solar plexus, which have been wide open, receptive and shooting energy out at great distances to other dancers and to audiences whilst we dance. The closing reverence brings our attention to our adjacent, personal human energy field, drawing distant energy connections back in to us. Like *closing the dancing book for the day*.

Whether you're a dancer or a teacher, if you simply walk out of the studio with energy centres wide open at the end of a high-power sequence or grand allegro section of class, you risk draining energy reserves and being overly exposed to whatever other energetic influences you may encounter in day-to-day life. Whatever style you dance in, consider reintroducing a calm, closing moment, a cooldown, a thank you or a reverence at the end of a session. Allow a yin moment of replenishing energy stores, draw the focus inwards towards your immediate energy field and gently take your attention to close each energy centre one after another to guard against vital energy loss or leakage. If the traditional thank you and gratitude to the teacher, musician or music of classical ballet and Eastern movement practice does not work in your dance context, then a quiet, personal thank you to your body for its focus and attention – a moment reaffirming the positive aspects of the training – is an equally effective closure to the efforts of daily practice.

Although our first objective here is to become aware of managing and balancing energy *in* motion whilst training or performing, in order to mitigate yin deficiency, we should not ignore possibilities to top up yin energy through recuperation activities after exertion. Much has been written about the need

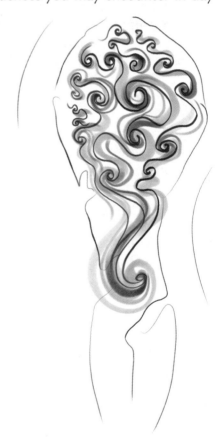

Figure 5.5   A closing ritual drawing energy down, away from the sensory organs, to store in the lower energy centre.

for recuperation after exercise (Dalleck n.d.). Activities such as sufficient deep sleep, massage, sauna and thermal bathing (Zar 2018); complementary movement forms such as yin yoga or other somatic practice (Alexander Technique, Feldenkrais Method, tai chi, chi kung) and meditation all have the ability to rebalance yin deficiency created from so much power-out, yang action. Other elements that are restorative, such as getting outdoors into nature and having other interests and hobbies outside the studio, are important to replenish and balance the hours focused on dance perfection. Some people may consider these activities less important than training itself or perhaps even consider them dispensable and simply *nice to do if you have the time*. However, in our quest for enhanced performance, they are as key to increasing power and stamina as the in-breath is to providing 'potential' when dancing.

ATTENTION IN MOTION

Focusing our mind and the process of filtering unhelpful attentional stimuli, although rarely addressed in dance, are central to assuring all aspects of our successful physical and mental performance, our energy renewal and our stamina. They are the keys that enable us to refine our practice and discover new heights of our personal best performance. We can all appreciate that in high-level sports, the difference between a winning athlete and those who did not quite make that level is not simply more muscles or more physical training or even more sport-specific knowledge, but it is their ability to manage their attentional process, their train of thought and their emotions in the moment, and to manage an unfaltering attentional focus.

When the mind is distracted the chi (energy) scatters. (Jahnke 2002, 37)

Unrelated trains of thought, self-talk and inner dialogue, however fleeting, drain energy and power from the system in the moment and shut down our capacity for sensory perception, undermining our best efforts and attempts to sustain our external attentional focus strategy. Developing our attention then means learning to consciously clear the mind of extraneous self-talk and commentaries, whether negative or positive, when we want optimal performance results. It's also the ability to recognize and nip unhelpful streams of thought in the bud in the moment and to be able to put them to one side and reset the mind with our chosen attentional focus.

Sport performance psychology typically involves techniques for developing attentional focus; quieting the mind; being 100 per cent in the moment in that one movement; performing without judgement, self-criticism and self-commentaries; and knowing one's performance strengths and building on those positives to form a foundational fabric for excellence. These concepts are often referred to as mindful practice and are based on Eastern movement practices' unified mind–body approach. They support the development of a desired no-mind, or clear mind, state. The ability to clear the mind of self-commentaries and of the desire to consciously interfere with one's physical performance and the ability to recognize and filter extraneous information and stimuli – the Eastern movement practice no-mind state – is advantageous for all activities. However, the physical and mental benefits promoted by this mindful practice increase, the more complex the movement challenge. This process of filtering, with the aid of an external attentional focus strategy as we saw in chapter 2, frees up cognitive reserves in the brain (Wulf 2007) and allows a heightened sensory perception and ability to respond in the moment. The Eastern movement practice of no-mind allows performers to be so present in the moment that they have the sensory capacity to detect an opponent's movement intention well before the opponent actually physically moves.

In Western dance practice, there is relatively little training time dedicated to integrated mind and attention strategies. These skills need to be developed as an integral element alongside the technical physical skills acquisition to support a complete mastery of performance. Ballet teacher Anna Paskevska highlights this process in ballet training and likens it to the Eastern training of samurai.

> For the dancer the process of reaching no-mind is repeated every day in class and in rehearsal. During the daily class, the dancer stands at the barre, her back is straight, her attention focused on performing each motion with utmost energy and accuracy. . . . In rehearsal, she learns the sequences, repeating the motions over and over until the actions flow within their own logical channels, unimpeded by conflicting thoughts. (Paskevska n.d., para. 13)

Developing our attentional focus and successfully filtering out unwanted thoughts and information in dance is just a learning process like any other (Taylor 2015). We start by simply becoming aware of our thinking processes and our attentional ability to stay focused. That's known as a metacognitive task, meaning we are going to think about the way we think! Here we are not concerned about *what* we are thinking. It's not about the content of the disruptive thoughts, but rather we observe the process of our thoughts and our attention to become aware of *how* we are thinking. It's not a question of trying to answer or to squash all of those passing questions or doubts that come up. They are a perfectly normal part of being sensitive and wanting to do your best; however, if they continually interrupt and disrupt your chosen external attention focus, then they are not supporting you to achieve your dancing best. Becoming aware of when your own train of thought interrupts your focus is the first step, followed by simple strategies that allow you to put thoughts to one side when they are not serving your best interests. Although dancers are very experienced at multitasking and processing large amounts of diverse input and information, we all perform best when using selective attention and minimum information in the moment for maximum cognitive and sensory capacity.

The good news is that our brain is infinitely adaptable. Although it takes conscious repetition to establish a new neural pathway when we first introduce a new way of thinking or approaching something, each time those neurons communicate with each other, that new neural pathway is strengthened, and the new process becomes more automatic and operates finally without

Attention and Focus in Practice

METACOGNITIVE AWARENESS

Dr Andrew McWilliams, psychiatrist, neuroscientist, dancer

We need to be aware that the artist is generally a different kind of person from a sportsperson, particularly dancers. Yes, they are dealing with the same technical, physical aspects, but actually the material is emotional, human material. The dancer is required to be a different kind of human being and have a disposition susceptible to emotional questions, to understanding something about the experience of humanity.

A sportsperson runs 100 metres and they are measured by a single metric – *time*. When you're a dancer, every moment of your performance is being measured and interpreted by an audience trying to understand something about who *you* are as a human being. So if you do a developpé à la seconde and your leg isn't as high as someone else's – it almost says something about who *you* are. It's not divorced from your body; it's actually a statement *about* your body. The work of the dancer is much more complex in terms of integrating, attending to and focusing on multiple different aspects. Try to understand and celebrate the difference between the things the dancer has to integrate. The dancer does need, though, to identify a strategy to start to manage the pull from all those different foci.

An 'inner dialogue' may be going on below the level of awareness. A dancer doing the Rose Adagio might be having some negative feelings about something that happened in class or perhaps something systemically going on in the company or even in her home life. If she is able to recognize that she is having these thoughts, in a metacognitive way, and start to sort of compartmentalize them, then that would be very helpful. The first step to doing that might be to be able to put them in 'a little box' somewhere for later. Having that kind of metacognitive awareness first, then taking action, would be exactly the thing that allows her to do well on stage.

conscious thought (Hani 2017). That's the reason that our habitual way of thinking or doing something appears so fixed, as if it were an integral part of who we *are*. It's simply that the pathway is so well used that it's always the fastest and most automatic route for our brain. The brain, however, remains adaptable at any age. No matter how experienced we are or how set in our ways, a conscious choice to try a new approach will create new pathways and new possibilities.

Let's take a look at a dance example from all the perspectives that we have touched on so far: energy, breath, mind, attentional focus and disruptive thoughts and self-talk. Imagine this example were in slow motion. We're in a sustained movement section and we've been successfully strong, stable and fluid using a new EF strategy to support a no-mind state: directing energy out through our movements in the desired direction and respecting the standing side for support, for example. Suddenly, we interrupt that focus because we remember that the next phrase coming up has a challenging technical element: a sustained balance and specific high leg line that we are a bit anxious about (disruptive, unhelpful thought). This cognitive interruption and self-related focus freezes our movement for an instant and we tense a little in anticipation. We shift from our chosen external focus a moment taking attention from the whole movement to focus on the specific control of the leg height (*where the mind will go, blood and energy will follow* [Quian 2017]). This attention shift drains power and stability from the whole and sends intention, energy and attention to the single body part, creating an energy dysfunction (IF, loss of stability, loss of power). We start to wobble as a result. A fleeting unhelpful thought and self-related commentary flashes through our mind, 'Umphf . . . I've never been good at balance'. We determine we had better revert to self-control (IF) as we have always done in challenging moments (well-established, old neural pathway) rather than trust the imagery we had rehearsed for this moment: *powerful roots going down and a precise, angled, high red line shooting out* (EF). We choose not to trust our body's superior, automatic capacities, and we give a conscious, extra push to the leg height at the expense of all other qualities (IF).

As a result, we grip all available muscles for stability, hold our breath and push the height of the leg. The balance is shaky, the energy flow inconsistent, the leg action heavy and muscular, and we can't hear the music. The execution is exhausting and not very successful. Before moving on to the next phrase, shaken and distracted, we conclude by reaffirming to ourselves, 'See! I'm useless at balance!' (reinforced old thought process and established neural pathway).

This sounds like a lot of attentional action, I know. However, all this and more takes place in a split second, and it's so easy to miss the process. It feels so normal, as if it were an invisible but parallel part of who you are. Once you begin to be conscious of the changes going on in your attentional focus and your self-talk or inner dialogue, you'll discover there is even more mental activity, more in and out of your desired focus than described in the previous example. Just a quick glance in the mirror is all it takes for a dancer to drop out of their desired attentional focus, diminishing performance and rendering it flat and two dimensional (Franklin 2014). Cathy Ward, former principal dancer of the Erick Hawkins Dance Company, observes that 'the dance ends (or is interrupted) when the attention (focus/awareness) drops. The dancer becomes like a flickering lamp, intermittently leaving the viewer in the dark' (Franklin 2014, xii).

From the perspective of Eastern movement practice, we aim to be functioning 100 per cent in the now, in this moment, in this movement. Whether our self-commentaries take us **backwards** into the past because we regret or are mad with ourselves for something that we did or did not do or we're anxious about something that has happened in the past or whether our self-commentaries project **forwards** into the future in the form of worries and 'What if?' dialogue with ourselves, energy is drained out of our system now. It is sucked backwards or forwards in the direction of our thoughts and our attention (see figure 5.6). *Where our mind will go, blood and energy follow* (Quian 2017). This attentional shift limits our ability to perceive and react in the moment. Our

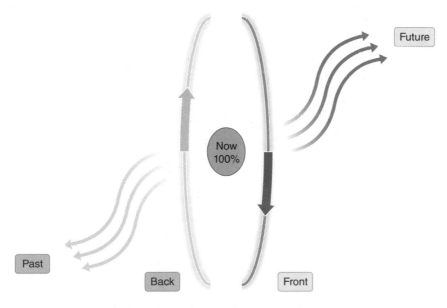

Figure 5.6   Past or future thoughts drain energy from the present moment.

ability to cultivate no-mind, then, *is* our ability to operate on maximum capacities with optimal power and energy right now. We often use the term to *pay* attention, and I like to imagine that: What we *pay* attention to has a definite *cost* and consequence on the quality of the present – so aim to *spend* wisely!

If you would like to begin to explore the process of your attention and thought patterns whilst dancing, start by tuning in from time to time during class. You might need to tell the teacher in confidence what you are doing because when you attempt this metacognitive practice of consciously observing your own thinking, you will not be 100 per cent present in your dance. Attentional shifts and self-talk often go on under the level of your awareness, so be patient with yourself as you try to identify your habitual attention process. If you are a dancer or a teacher, the content of the focus and the inner self-talk might be different, but the exercise of observing the process is the same.

EXPLORATION 5.5 – BRINGING ATTENTION TO THE PROCESS OF ATTENTION

Start by observing your attention and its habitual shifts at the beginning of class when the exercises are a little less challenging. Have your journal close by so that you can jot down your observations after an exercise. Some exercises or dance contexts might provoke more self-talk and more distractions or shifts of attention than others. Can you notice when your attention shifts most frequently? More at the barre and less in the centre? When you do controlled sustained adage or when you have to memorize a lot of new choreography? Is it different on different days according to external influences or your mood or emotional state? Can you make a correlation between your mood or emotional state and the frequency of attentional shifts or unhelpful thought interruptions so that you can identify areas that need the most support?

If you want to track your development, use the questions and suggested scoring examples in table 5.2 to help develop your awareness. After an exercise or after class, give yourself a score for the amount of time you felt you were able to stay in the moment and in the movement, in a no-mind state or with your chosen external attentional focus. The example in the table is 50 per cent of the time during the exercise. That's a pretty good score.

Remember your objective is to identify what's going on and what your typical attention and thinking pattern is whilst dancing. You're not trying to solve everything at once, just to bring your attention to your attention.

TABLE 5.2   Developing the Process of Attention: Simple Attention Observation Examples

ATTENTION	EXAMPLE	SCORE	OTHER OBSERVATIONS (e.g., Which exercise? What context? Emotion or mood today? Other factors)
Per cent of time spent in chosen external attentional focus or foci	Feeling two-way pull, delicate unfolding last few centimetres, push the floor away, feel the touch of the retiré (EF)	50%	
Number of times attention shifted to body part or self-adjustment	Pull in my stomach, straighten the leg, point the foot, wrap and hold glutes and legs to balance (IF)	4	
Number of thought interruptions	'This teacher is always quiet. I wonder what she thinks about my . . .' 'Agh. I've no power in my legs today.' 'I never have high legs. It's so depressing.' 'Actually, that balance didn't look too bad.' 'No! Pirouettes next up.' 'Ough! I shouldn't have eaten so much.'	6	
Reset mind	Give yourself a score today on a scale of 1 to 10. How successfully were you able to put thoughts to one side to refocus and reset your chosen attentional foci?	5/10	

Once you begin the process of observing your attention and thought processes, you might become conscious of the *content* of some of your self-talk, inner dialogue or interruptions, particularly if the content tends to be self-critical or negative. The sensitive, conscientious and sometimes perfectionist nature of many dancers means that we are experts at self-criticism. We usually identify with great facility everything that is *lacking* in our performance and about ourselves and typically have a long mental list of the aspects that still need work (Harari 2018). Our self-critical neural pathways are well trodden! However, these critical thoughts and negative self-observations are rarely factual. You can spot these thought patterns easily because they frequently contain words such as *always*, *never*, *ever* and *worst* or involve *should*, *must* and *ought* instructions. This critical propensity can make it challenging to move on from these debilitating patterns and begin to build strong performance foundations that acknowledge our existing strengths and positive qualities. These critical observation skills have supported us this far in our dancing journey; however, with constant repetition, these well-worn pathways become paralyzing and now hold us back from reaching another performance level (Bradberry 2014).

One simple technique to quiet the mind is to take your attention to any of your five senses (EF) to dispel disruptive thought. This brings you back instantly into the moment, into your movement, like with the breath (as mentioned in the following attention and focus in practice by Dr Gay Watson), at any point. Place your attention on your sense of touch, on the sounds, on what you see, on what you smell and, why not, on what you taste. When you create your safe place (Watson's attention and focus in practice), the more sensory details you can recall, the more real it can be, the more effective it will be at

---

Attention and Focus in Practice

DISPERSING CRITICAL THOUGHT

Dr Gay Watson, specialist in Eastern philosophy, psychotherapist, teacher, author

Paying attention to the way we habitually pay attention, this is the way we learn these new skills. The most important is to notice when it's happening and that it *is* happening and then not continue with the narrative. You can label them 'unhelpful thought' or 'critical thought'. When you have an unhelpful thought, 'I'm looking fatter than ever', just notice it, 'OK, there it goes again. Critical thought!' But don't continue the story, 'Oh, I can't do it. I'm an awful person! I mustn't eat so much!' If you say 'Oh, critical thought', you cut it off. Go back to the breath. Go back to the movement you are doing. Critical thought gets fed by the story. Gradually, you won't go there quite so much. It's like mowing over a patch of weeds an awful lot. Gradually, they don't grow up; they lose energy. It's the same process. It sounds easy and we all know it's incredibly challenging, but it's just the same as learning a new technique in dance.

Go back to the breath. When you pay attention to your breath, in one nano-second you bring mind and body together. Mostly our minds and our bodies are incredibly split. The mind is often off doing all sorts of things and deeply divorced from the body. When you place your attention on your breath, then you're back in your sensations, with your experience, and you're grounded.

If it all becomes a bit too much, you can create a safe place where you can go. Choose a memory where you felt really good doing something you love or with someone – a family member or a pet even. It could be a physical sensation where you feel good. Stop the story and go to your safe place. If we can have some happy thoughts and a good place to go, it produces oxytocin and you feel better. Whereas critical thought is like a little poison drip.

dissipating critical thought. So, if your safe place is at the beach, for example, then ask yourself What do I hear? Can I hear the water? Can I hear the birds or distant cries of people playing? Can I feel the sand under my feet? What temperature is the sand? How does the beach smell (Foong n.d.)?

As we quiet the 'thinking' brain, clear the mind and make space by moving our attention to the senses, a whole chain reaction of healing occurs in the body. Energy flows, power surges, breathing deepens, pulse lowers, serotonin (our natural antidepressor) is produced, anxiety reduces (because of lower levels of cortisol and adrenalin) and attention itself is heightened. This global response to a small shift of attention enables enhanced learning, creativity and artistry.

It could be groundbreaking to create a foundation for yourself that acknowledges your strengths and your dance accomplishments. Shift focus away from some of the inevitable, critical self-observations to introduce a few positives. Cultivating an attitude of positive gratitude and thanks towards yourself (and others) is shown scientifically to reduce anxiety and increase energy levels (Bradberry 2017). As a starting point for your positive foundation, take a moment and write down at least half a dozen skills, qualities or things you do well already in dance and that you appreciate about yourself. You may struggle at first to find six aspects, not because this is factual, but simply because it's not a thought process you have developed yet. Be patient as you create new pathways. These could be things that you have already

Attention and Focus in Practice

POSITIVE THOUGHT TRANSLATES TO THE WHOLE SPECTRUM

Kailey Kaba, professional ballet dancer, Finnish National Ballet

I wish I would have kept my confidence early on – been open to changing, yes, but not lost myself. This put me into a downward spiral of second-guessing my choices, and when you start to doubt yourself, it's impossible to move forward. For me, my injuries have come when I doubted myself, had a fear of not meeting my own and others' expectations. It created a negative self-talk, 'I can't do it. No, no, what if this happens?' You know your inside voices can get the best of you sometimes. Of course, when you're on pointe, turning and afraid that you're going to fall or slip, then an extra wobble is already being created. It's really the power of thought, but then that's for anything! Creating positive thought and positive things in your life translates to the whole spectrum.

mentally ticked off as accomplished such as a beautiful, lyrical quality in adage, speed and attack in small jumps and comfortable double pirouette. Or they might be qualities that seem to come naturally, such as a developed musicality or good kinaesthetic memory for choreography. Have the list to hand, take it to class and rehearsals with you and reread it at least once per day like an affirmation to consciously build a positive foundational fabric. Actively seek to add to the list other positive qualities, skills or accomplishments. I give you the challenge to aim for about 30 positive things on your list by the time you finish this book. You could add to your reflective journal other positive, life-affirming sayings that you come across that resonate with you. Find a daily, positive saying to start the morning with your breakfast, like taking a vitamin supplement for the mind. Trust that these positive affirmations work at a quantum level, weaving their way into your being like a gossamer net that supports and creates new pathways in the brain and body, effecting change slowly but surely, drop by drop, in our energy field, in our chemistry (Wulf and Lewthwaite 2016) and in our very cells.

A Dancer's Daily Affirmation

Fill every cell in my body with spirit, light and love

Let me hear the quiet voice of knowing

Let me distinguish from the voice of my fears

Let my fears not have authority over me

Let me trust in my path and in my process

Although I may not know where I am going or why

I place myself in the universe's hands

And release the need to control the outcome

Let me work through a clear head, a clear heart, and a clear body

Thank you for this moment

Thank you for the access to the wisdom

Thank you for this body

Inspired by the teachings of Caroline Myss.

REFLECTION PROMPTS

- Looking at table 5.1, can you brainstorm a few of the most obvious yin moments in your dance style? Are there examples that you could easily begin to focus more on in your training to replenish energy?

- What words or images did you use to describe the sensations you felt during the sacrum or occipital breathing exercise in explorations 5.4*a* and 5.4*b*? Be sure to have those words somewhere to hand to refer to as you begin to develop more of the yin elements of your dance practice. Just one of the words or images will be enough to trigger and enable the same beneficial sensations *whilst* you are dancing.

- What did you learn about your attentional focus process in class in the self-observation task (exploration 5.5)? Did you notice moments or exercises where you experienced more frequent interruptions? Or moments or exercises where you were able to sustain your attention better? Dr Andrew McWilliams suggests putting thoughts and worries to one side in 'a box' to deal with at another appropriate moment. Do you have another creative image for putting disruptive dialogue to one side for later?

- What sort of personal thank you, closing ritual or reverence can you imagine creating for your daily dance practice? It can be a silent or inner ritual or affirmation that you do whilst stretching at the end of class so that no one else is aware of it.

I've shared for inspiration the Dancer's Daily Affirmation that I created and use for myself every day whilst stretching after dancing. What's important is that the words or images are personal and meaningful to you.

PART II

CUEING ATTENTION

CHAPTER 6

TEACHING WITH EXTERNAL ATTENTIONAL FOCUS

When you adopt an external focus, you enhance all simultaneously: power, precision and artistry. You never have to negate the importance or the necessity of technique for the sake of artistry.

Raymond Chai (2019)

*C*hoosing to harness the benefits of an external attentional focus and integrate attention and focus strategies into your teaching practice is a gradual process. It starts by simply developing awareness of how you currently teach and cue and what your own go-to control approach is.

Both an internal focus approach on body parts and an external focus on the movement effect are potential movement control approaches. Both have the same original intention to facilitate skills learning, refine motor control and enhance performance results. (Refer to table 2.1 for descriptions of internal and external focus of attention.) If you habitually use or were taught primarily through an internal focus approach, as many of us were, then the consistent intensity of effort this demands and the frequency of conscious interference with the movement will feel normal to you. In this case, IF control instructions will naturally surface quickest when you give feedback in teaching because they are the most familiar to you and have the most well-trodden neural pathways. In teaching, just like with parenting, unless we make a conscious choice to do it differently, we are likely to teach exactly as *we* ourselves were taught.

Changing a lifelong habit and replacing it with a new habit involves cognitive effort and commitment at first; however, seeing immediate returns in terms of students' improved physical and mental performance, attention to learning and speed of grasping new skills and their renewed enjoyment of their dance practice consistently reaffirms this new choice. In no time, it becomes more fluent and a more automatic go-to response when giving instruction or feedback. Whatever your own dance expertise and specialism, you will experience a sense of increased effectiveness in your teaching delivery, and not only your students but also you will enjoy a sense of reduced effort and renewed energy in class.

Today's dancers and teachers are perhaps the first generation to choose the metacognitive task of developing awareness of *how* they learn and teach. Embarking on the task of unlearning a habitual movement control approach and consciously introducing an alternative way of approaching movement learning is a double task. Imagine that subsequent generations will not have to undertake this double effort of unlearning one way of working and adopting a new approach in midcareer. For dancers who have already trained with their attention on the effect of the movement (EF) since a young age, it feels completely normal for them to use mindful techniques as a control strategy for movement.

The current predominance of an IF control approach in Western dance teaching is perhaps also a generational phenomenon. In my own experience, some of the older generation of teachers seemed to use fewer words when teaching and used an external approach more frequently. Perhaps this generational difference is due in part to increased teacher knowledge today and the emphasis in Western dance on achieving certain extreme physical goals. Perhaps there is more requirement for conformity in dance today. This has led, as in sports practice, to the mistaken assumption that more self-related, conscious control would be beneficial in order to achieve these increased demands. Perhaps in previous generations there was more time and space for the development of self-knowledge, implicit learning and individuality. Some older-generation ballet teachers also simply taught using the original French terminology that describes, for the most part, the form, the quality and the outcome of the movements (EF). This means that an external focus of attention was somehow built into the original classical vocabulary and that their classes almost exclusively promoted an external focus of attention without the teachers being aware of its benefits or indeed actually consciously choosing this as a movement control approach.

The good news is that many teachers today, like professional dancers in the study (Guss-West and Wulf 2016), are still using an external focus of attention intuitively for some of their teaching feedback and instructions. To develop the use of EF systematically as a strategy in your teaching practice, start by identifying which types of EF you *already* use regularly in class (figure 2.3) and then gradually look for opportunities to introduce *more* of something that you are already doing.

We can also begin by modifying the body part–related instructions (IF) that we might habitually use whilst teaching by making a small shift in our choice of wording. A quick win that takes little effort at first is to simply omit references to a body part in your instructions whenever possible. If you are demonstrating, having a student demonstrate or even just using your hands to represent the action, then you are already giving enormous amounts of EF information regarding the form, the quality of the movement and your teaching priorities. For example, teaching the action of a developpé, or an unfolding leg, you might add to your demonstration the description 'unfolding and reaching through' rather than 'unfolding the leg and reaching through the foot'. The 'missing' body-part information is not necessary when supported visually by demonstration. In attention and focus workshops, I make a fun activity out of this first awareness-building step for teachers and ask them to teach colleagues a basic movement without naming a body part. Their colleagues imitate the buzzer sound of a TV game show every time one of them uses a body-part reference. This immersion activity provokes a lot of laughter and silliness; however, teachers report that this simple game helps them to become conscious of their own use of instructions and feedback and their choice of cueing vocabulary, and to this day a buzzer goes off in their head and a smile crosses their face each time they name a body part in class.

This first quick-win action might make us focus only on what we *can't* say as we begin to omit body-part references from our teaching, a bit like we feel when we decide to become vegan and then we focus only on all the ingredients we *can't* use in our cooking! As you become more conscious of your habitual choices, however, you can shift your focus and gradually become more cre-ative while exploring all the rich, EF alternative 'ingredients', possibilities and combinations until you become expert at creative EF 'cooking' alternatives that can address even the most subtle of feedback necessities.

EXTERNAL FOCUS FOR ENHANCED LEARNING

The fascinating findings of research on adopting an external attentional focus extend beyond the immediate benefits to performance and demonstrate that learning itself is likewise significantly affected. The speed of mastering motor skills is increased, the recall of learning is enhanced and long term and permanent changes to movement skills are all evidenced benefits of implementing an external focus of attention strategy in teaching. These benefits are consistent across different movement contexts and at all skills levels. Adopting an external focus control approach as a systematic teaching strategy will promote effective outcomes whether we are teaching initial movement skills, the mastering of technique for vocational students, the refining of movement with professionals or working with movement rehabilitation and injury or facilitating movement for senior populations and those with special movement challenges.

The learning process has been categorized into three basic learning phases (Fitts 1964), and learners are seen to move from an initial cognitive phase, through an associative phase and eventually reach an autonomous phase of movement. The initial *cognitive phase*, as the term suggests, demands a lot of thinking about how the movement should work and a lot of self-talk. Learners tend initially to focus on the sequence of the individual component elements of the movement and the coordination of their body parts. As a result of this conscious body-part control, the movement of the first phase is slow, inconsistent and inefficient. It requires large amounts of energy and muscular recruitment and typically engages muscle groups irrelevant to the task. The *associative phase* is an intermediary phase where, with practice, performance becomes more consistent, inefficiency is reduced and at least some aspects of the movement can be executed automatically. In the final phase, the *autonomous phase*, movements become efficient, accurate and consistent and, ideally, controlled autonomously by our body's fast reflexive movement response with little conscious cognitive activity. This allows free attentional capacity for other aspects of performance and artistic expression in the case of dance.

The emphasis of the initial cognitive learning phase concerns a focus on the form of the movement and on acquiring basic skills; however, the interpretation of how best to achieve that skills-focused learning objective seems to provoke different responses from teachers. Many hold to the belief that to break down a movement in initial skills learning, it's essential to draw learners' attention to the conscious control of their own body parts, as Dr Gabriele Wulf mentions in the foreword. Is this really the most effective learning path to successfully acquire the initial movement skills? Research suggests not. As with all other skills levels, drawing a learner's attention to self-related conscious control blocks efficient, fluid movement. It slows the rate of learning and of reaching the autonomous phase of movement relative to the alternative of encouraging a focus on the desired effect of the movement (EF). (See figure 6.1.) However we were taught initial movement skills, these robust scientific findings hold true and can be valuably harnessed and integrated into teaching practice to increase teaching efficiency.

One example of the many research studies particularly relevant to dance was conducted with young gymnasts of 12 years of age (Abdollahipour et al. 2014). The study involved a half-turn jump with the requirement to demonstrate a precise, correct landing position. The research measured, therefore, not just the immediate effect of attentional focus on jump height but also its impact on mastering correct movement form. The internal focus instruction was to 'focus on the direction that the *hands* point after the half-turn jump', and the external focus instruction was to 'focus on the direction that the *sticker* (on the chest) points after the half-turn jump'. The benefits of the EF trials to jump height were confirmed, as they had been in multiple other jump height research studies; however, the study also confirmed the impact of an EF approach versus an IF approach in relation to mastering the correct movement form. In the study, points were deducted for incorrect landing positions. By using the sticker as a teaching resource (EF), not only was the jump height superior but the landing position and the form of the movement were also 50 per cent more accurate in the EF trials than those of the IF trials in which the attention was drawn to the hands. This means that the rate of learning was also enhanced through the use of an external focus of attention.

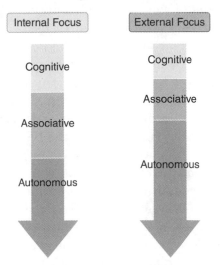

Figure 6.1   The impact of an external focus of attention on the speed of learning.

Adapted from G. Wulf, *Attention and Motor Skills Learning* (Champaign, IL: Human Kinetics, 2007), 3.

Choosing to adopt an external focus of attention is a more effective and more economical teaching strategy, and reduces significantly the need for teacher feedback, demonstration and repetition. EF feedback not only affects immediate learning and performance but also promotes long-term learning changes to movement skills and significantly improves later recall of movement details (Wulf 2013).

These long-term benefits are measured by retention tests in which participants return to the same movement task several days later and are asked to repeat the task with no further instructions. Depending on the study, performance accuracy, precision, quality of movement or capacity for microadjustment (balance) are measured. Those who learnt using an external focus of attention consistently excelled in the retention of skills learning, often improving on their last measured performance, indicating an embodiment and consolidation of learning and a permanent change to the movement skill. Skills learnt with an external focus appear to be embodied to such an extent that they are transferable to new, more demanding learning contexts (Wulf 2013). Significant for learning dance skills, research shows that the more challenging the movement task, the more pronounced are the benefits of adopting an external focus of attention. It's even more important to resist the temptation to revert to self-related control precisely when addressing more complex movement challenges (Wulf, Töllner and Shea 2007).

There is a common misunderstanding, in my experience, regarding the potential range and subtlety of using an external focus of attention in teaching. Some teachers imagine that EF is useful only as general or global motivational feedback: 'reaching for the stars' to promote a general extension of the movement or 'exploding like a firework' to create the dynamic, multidimensional expansion of a movement. Breaking down the small component parts of a movement for beginners during initial skills learning or focusing on the quality of small technical details whilst refining movement for more advanced students can all be successfully addressed by using the different types of EF (figure 2.3) and by modifying the wording of habitual instructions. EF cues can be crafted to address microtechnical detail, subtle movement quality or anatomical precision.

With beginners, tangible, proximal EF such as dance clothes, props, stickers and other teaching resources, the floor, the barre and a partner dancer are readily accessible foci to choose from. You might use instructions such as reach through your *shoes*, stretch your *tights or leggings*, focus on drawing *a circle* with *your prop*. When considering using imaginary EF in class, research suggests that whilst all skills levels can benefit from the application of imagery, the ability to purposefully apply subtle metaphorical imagery involving multisensory layers is a learnt ability. This ability seems to develop in parallel with skills development (Nordin and Cumming 2007; Pavlik and Nordin-Bates 2016). The extensive use of imagery for refining movement quality is more appropriate for advanced students (Pavlik and Nordin-Bates 2016).

Sensory EF, touch and imagery can be the most easily adapted for microdetailed, refining feedback with more advanced students. In looking to enhance movement quality in the unfolding leg, or developpé (figure 6.2), we could draw the student's attention to focus on the quality of the last few centimetres of the journey or to feel the continuous spiral of the unfolding or to imagine the action unfolding like a leaf bud. To achieve the desired spacious couronne, or fifth position of the arms in a port de bras, we might ask the student to create maximum space within the circle, or we could ask students to imagine containing dancing energy while we support this with a visual teaching gesture. We could also use touch and place our hands gently on the shoulders with a 'roll and down the back' movement intention. The possibilities are infinite. The choice of EF is open to exploration according to individual teacher and student preferences and the teaching context.

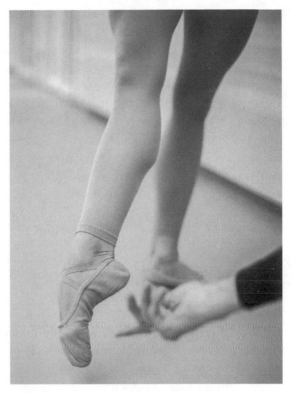

Figure 6.2   Refining movement details using an imaginary external focus of attention – unfolding like a leaf. (Tchri and Clare)

EXPLORING POTENTIAL EXTERNAL FOCUS TYPES FOR TEACHING

Choosing appropriate modes of EF feedback is not a matter of one-size-fits-all, nor is it a question of teacher preference. Although it's a challenging belief to let go of, teaching research confirms that just because certain imagery or certain kinds of proprioceptive feedback worked for us, that does not mean that they will therefore be the most effective feedback for other learners. For example, research demonstrates that when using EF imagery, the student's *feelings* towards the image will affect the movement outcome (Pavlik and

Nordin-Bates 2016). To maximize our teaching efficiency and facilitate our choice of EF amidst the range of possibilities, we could consider selecting EF types according to the learning styles of our individual students.

A student's **learning style** refers to the way different learners receive and share learning information most efficiently. The basic learning styles are defined as visual (representations, diagrams), aural or auditory (sounds, talking), read and write (words, text), kinaesthetic (perception, sensory, practice) and multimodal (varying according to the learning context and includes several or all modes in order for the learner to achieve a 360-degree understanding). These are referred to as the VARK learning styles and all of the styles can be addressed successfully through the choice of different external focus types (Fleming and Mills 1992; Vark Learn n.d.; University of Iowa 2006). See table 6.1 near the end of this chapter.

THE TEACHER AS AN EFFECTIVE EXTERNAL FOCUS

It's worth remembering that *we* are in fact the most effective external focus teaching resource available for students (figure 6.3). We provide a multimodal external focus of attention that addresses different learning styles. We can provide these external foci:

- Visually with the clothes and the colours that we choose to wear. This choice immediately reflects appropriate presentation and transmits a desired physical tension and posture. Clothes can be used to draw the learner's attention to priority learning elements such as our clear line, our verticality or the part of the clothing that is leading the move- ment – zips, waist bands, logos, patterns or colours. With special needs groups you want to be easily identifiable, so you might wear a bright colour or wear bright socks or shoes if you want to highlight the actions of your feet.

- Visually through demonstration. We transmit not only the obvious content and form of the movement, but we also equally provide a 'hologram' of other information: the desired movement quality; our movement priorities; our intention; appropriate effort, breath, energy flow, mental approach, mindset; and our emotions. *How* we transmit that information is a much more powerful teaching EF than simply the content itself.

- Aurally by the use of our voice, which is a versatile EF. We can draw attention to the learning priorities with the creative use of the voice: to the musicality and to the rhythm and accents by using a sing- song voice. We can use sounds that describe the desired quality of the movement, we can transmit the appropriate breath or we can

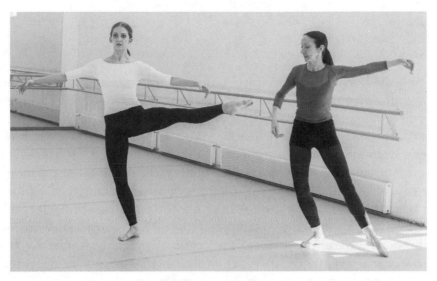

Figure 6.3   The teacher as an effective external attentional focus –
sending energy out through the hand and beyond to the sunlight. (Kailey
and Clare)

provide an EF simply by drawing students' attention to the sound of
our words.

Thanks to the functioning of mirror neurons, we teach 360 degrees of
information constantly simply by being and breathing and dancing with the
students and dancers. If there is a disconnect between what we *say* and how
we act or how we *are*, it is the *how* we are and *how* we approach the movement
ourselves that will transmit to the dancers through the mirror neuron system
and via kinaesthetic learning in both class and rehearsal contexts.

The human mirror system enables us to share another person's intention
and emotion by observing their gaze, posture, breathing and physical tension. (Karin and Nordin-Bates 2019, 5)

A teacher came hurriedly to see me after an attentional focus workshop
with her young classical ballet students. In the workshop, we had been taking
our attention to the potential use of the breath to enhance movement outcome. She excitedly shared with me, 'That's so fantastic thank you to see
them listening and breathing in this way this morning it's really transformed
their dancing I'm so happy to see that *finally* it's so strange I don't understand
because I've been telling them and telling them breathe breathe for the last
couple of years but you know they just don't listen! (Gasp for breath.)' I smiled
and breathed calmly with her a moment. We have to *be* the change we wish
to see from our students. They will pick up by transmission *how* we are and
how we approach movement, not *what* we say.

USING TOUCH AS AN EFFECTIVE EXTERNAL FOCUS

Directing the learner's attention to a specific touch point to communicate learning information is an extremely effective and efficient EF teaching tool that is already commonly used in dance practice. Touch is particularly appropriate for the kinaesthetic-style learner. With a specific gesture, we draw the learner's attention to the sensation of the touch point – to the sensation of the pressure, the lightness, the warmth, the quality, the direction or the intention of the touch. Teaching time spent using touch as a teaching tool is time well spent because the touch provides multiple future feedback opportunities. Touch promotes an immediate response to the direct information transmitted in that moment: the appropriate effort, tension, resistance, softening, breath and flow of energy. Later on, there are infinite further possibilities because the touch point also provides a lasting, holographic imprint of all this information. This information can easily be referenced and recalled at any moment during movement by the dancers themselves or prompted by a simple visual or verbal cue from the teacher. As you perhaps experienced during explorations 5.4*a* and 5.4*b*, when you take your attention to the sacrum or the occipital area, the sensation of the pressure and the warmth of your partner's hands seem present to this day. In my direct experience, the information transmitted through touch is lasting and easily accessible to the dancer at any point whilst moving as a multidimensional, proprioceptive impression.

Using touch effectively requires that we focus our attention on exactly what we are trying to communicate through the touch and how. With learning information gathered through the senses, we know that it is the quality of the touch that is the most important rather than the quantity (Bannon and Holt 2012). The use of touch in Western dance teaching can be arbitrary. It's often fleeting, and its desired message is sometimes ambiguous, which wastes a teaching opportunity because the dancers are unable to effectively learn from it. In my own early classical training, for example, the teacher inadvertently communicated her frustration and what seemed, at my young age, like anger through her touch, which reinforced a sense of inadequacy as fingernails dug in and turnout was forced with inappropriate tension. My multisensory recall is vivid to this day; sensory feedback never leaves the learner. There is a growing consciousness in some countries and cultures today of the need to actively seek the permission of the receiver or learner in order to use touch in teaching practice. Because touch is such an effective teaching tool in movement skills learning, it would be a great shame to avoid using it simply because of a lack of a clear protocol (Assandri 2019; Outevsky 2013).

It's important then that we attend to the information we *actually* want to transmit and aim to make it very clear. We then actively seek the permission of the receiver, engage their attention and draw their focus to the touch to acknowledge the transmission of information and to consolidate the learning. Many dance teachers successfully seek that permission by asking briefly 'May I show you?' or 'I'd like to show you where . . .' or 'I'd like to show you how that might feel. Are you ok with that?'

For the effective use of touch in dance teaching and maximum learning, I adopt some of the basic protocols that a therapist would use because therapists use touch extensively in their work to diagnose, communicate, treat and give feedback and instructions. Consider the following when using touch as an EF feedback choice in dance:

- **Information** – Be clear and ask yourself what you want to transmit with your hands.

- **Quality** – Consider the timing of your gesture, the quality, the pressure, the direction and the intention.

- **Gesture** – Choose an appropriate gesture. Is it a one- or two-finger touch point to provide a focal point and draw the attention (figure 6.4), flat fingers with even pressure to encourage a reaction, a whole hand for directional information, two hands for dynamic relational information? Perhaps you spontaneously use some other body part: your elbow, knee, foot. Is it an appropriate body part to transmit the desired information? Ask yourself how is it perceived by the receiver?

- **External attention** – Guide the receiver's attention to the touch by asking a question such as 'Can you feel the pressure, direction or quality of the touch?' Or give an instruction such as 'Press against my hand', 'Breathe into my hand', 'Focus on the warmth' or 'Focus on the touch point'.

- **Eye contact** – Seek eye contact to assess the receiver's comfort level and understanding.

- **Timing** – Sustain the touch long enough. It takes time for the receiver to identify and register the touch and to comprehend the information being transmitted and for the neural networks, fascia and muscles to respond to that information. Physical therapists typically sustain a touch a minimum of three breaths to achieve that response. If sustaining for three breath cycles is not appropriate in the context then sustain the touch at least for a slow count of three to allow time for that body–brain–body journey.

- **Test** – If you are unsure of your skill at using touch, a good strategy as a teacher is to ask the receiver or learner 'What did you feel or understand?' This gives you valuable feedback about the effectiveness of your use of touch and also consolidates the learning for the receiver.

Touch can be used as an effective EF to enhance movement outcome whether you as the teacher are providing the touch-based feedback or whether it is used in a specific guided-touch exercise between students or peers. Involving peers in an EF touch exercise promotes implicit learning and provides efficient teaching. The 'active dancers' providing the touch are actively learning just as much about movement problem solving and what creates a successful movement and focus of attention as the 'receiving dancer'.

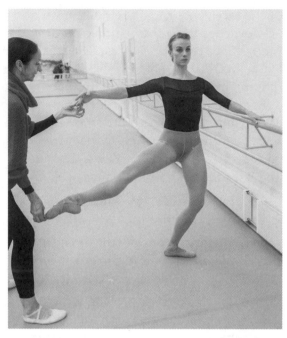

Figure 6.4   Using two-finger touch as an effective external focus to draw attention to the relationship between two distant focal points. (Clare and Tehri)

Those that have learnt implicitly are less dependent on verbal–analytical processes to support performance, so [display] greater neural efficiency. (Masters 2014)

In a simple, free exploration for enhanced balance (figure 6.5), Ben and Tehri (active) provide Kailey (receiving) with a clear, firm, two-finger touch point on either side of the arm just above the wrist joint. They are not supporting Kailey's weight nor leading or promenading her. Their role is to provide a consistent pressure and touch point reference and to flow and follow the improvisation of Kailey as best they can. I ask the active dancers to provide the slightest outward traction so that the receiver feels a gentle, even pull across the chest but otherwise to simply follow the movements that she can sustain in her second position. Kailey focuses in the two directions of the touch points simultaneously and allows energy to flow out horizontally from the heart energy centre, through the touch points and beyond as far as her attention will permit. Using only this focus of attention, the receiving dancer improvises a promenade of alternating fast and slow balances forwards or backwards. They explore their own ability to sustain the focus of attention whilst enjoying the enhanced stability and the improved, automatic microadjustments to balance promoted by the EF (Wulf 2013). Active and receiving rotate so that all students get to experience each role and sense directly and implicitly how a shift of attention or distraction that takes the focus from the EF back onto the self has an immediate detrimental effect on consistency, strength and balance.

This is an exploration that might take 10 minutes of class time; however, the impression of the touch points is embedded and becomes a lasting teaching tool. The objective of the exploration is to move straight on and immediately repeat the balance improvisation individually, using only the recall of the touch points as the focus of attention. Taking their attention to the recall of the touch points, dancers discover that they are not dependent on others and can enjoy the same enhanced stability by using their own recall, as with real partners.

'Interactive learning triples students' gains in knowledge', declares Harvard active learning specialist Eric Mazur (Lambert 2012, para. 9). 'Active learners take new information and *apply* it, rather than merely taking note of it. First-hand use of new material develops personal ownership' (Lambert 2012, para. 14). Mazur's approach teaches through questioning rather than teaching by telling (Mazur 2009).

In another effective peer exploration, students use touch to promote the simultaneous extension of the five lines of the arabesque out into space. We frequently see dancers who construct their arabesque mentally in separate pieces or body parts. Even if there is only a millisecond of separation between the parts, we can identify the steps: first the arms, then the leg, then the demi-pointe and last, reaching through the crown. This construction in parts uses multiple movement units and makes achieving a successful dynamic balance or a clear, expressive movement challenging. By taking a dancer's attention

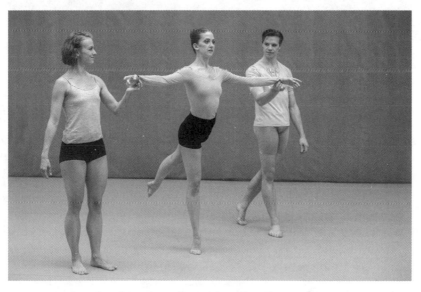

Figure 6.5   Using partner touch as an effective external focus during an exploration in balance enhancement. (Kailey with Tehri and Ben)

to five touch points that will become the five arabesque lines, we promote a global, cohesive view of the movement. The lines extend out as one whole brush stroke, like the striking of a match, and the arabesque is transformed (figures 6.7a-c).

EXPLORATION 6.1 – USING PEER TOUCH POINTS IN ARABESQUE

This exploration involves groups of six students who rotate roles so that each one has the opportunity to be the receiver of the touch points. Each of the five active dancers establish one touch point after another whilst the receiving dancer stands in a relaxed arabesque line à terre (on the floor) (figures 6.6 and 6.7a).

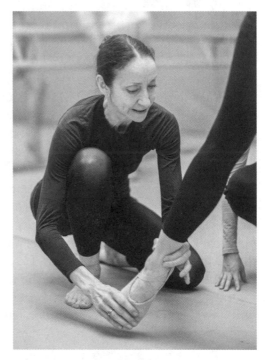

Figure 6.6   Using touch as an effective external focus, an active dancer establishes one of the five focal touch points for the arabesque. (Clare)

- The three active dancers providing touch points on the arms and the arabesque playing leg give an even pressure using the thumb and the index or middle finger on each side of the limb just above the ankle or the wrist joint. They exert the slightest traction outwards in the direction of the line. The active dancer on the playing leg gives the suggestion of a lengthening away with the traction rather than an upwards motion (figures 6.6 and 6.7a).

- The active dancer drawing attention to the supporting side, or roots of the arabesque, gives a firm, calm downward pressure into the ground with two hands to encourage the stability and downward extension (figure 6.7a).

- The active dancer drawing attention to the crown extension cups the occipital bone and uses the thumb and index or middle finger to provide two touch points on either side of the bony process behind the ears and exerts a gentle upward traction. They check that the receiving dancer can still freely move their head and that there is no holding (figure 6.7a).

As in the improvised balance exploration, the active dancers are not supporting or controlling. They are simply drawing the receiver's attention to their pressure.

Ask the receiving dancer if they can feel the five focal touch points in the five directions. Is the pressure from all five about the same? Is there too much or too little traction in one direction? (See figures 6.5, 6.6 and 6.7a.)

To coordinate all the active dancers in the arabesque, I ask the receiver to make space and draw breath in over three slow counts whilst I count out loud. With the sustained out-breath, the receiving dancer extends simultaneously in the direction of each of the five touch points and beyond as far as their attention can go. Active dancers dissolve away in the direction of the extension with the receiving dancers' out-breath, giving space (figures 6.7b and 6.7c). Any brusque movement of the active dancers or movement contrary to the line of the energy flow they are encouraging in the arabesque will draw the receiving dancer off balance.

The arabesque continues to expand and curve away, seemingly effortlessly and endlessly in the five directions with the out-breath in a constant, expansive curve of minimum muscular effort (figure 6.7c). Natural breathing can resume and continue throughout the sustain without disturbing the arabesque, provided that the attention remains clearly on the direction of the five focal touch points and the extending lines.

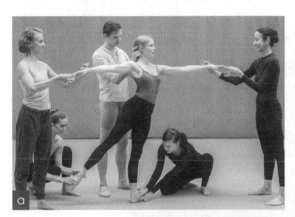
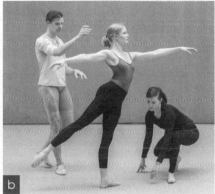
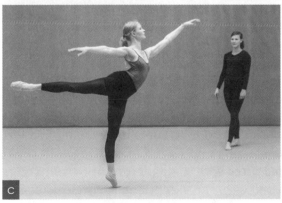

Figure 6.7   Using peer touch as an effective external focus in arabesque to produce a global movement cohesion – (a) establishing focal touch points for the five directions, (b) active dancers dissolve away and give space, (c) receiving dancer extends in all five directions into arabesque. (Emmi with Tehri, Kailey, Ben, Johanna and Clare)

All participants are actively learning in this exploration and developing awareness of the process of focusing attention and the five simultaneous directions. Active dancers can sense immediately the receiving dancer who resists the gentle traction and the direction of the movement. They can feel the receiving dancer who habitually initiates the movement with a body-part focus because they tend to contract and pull inwards, away from the direction of their peers in an attempt to regain conscious control of their movement. And they can feel through their touch those who focus on the lift of the playing or gesture leg with a muscle-led initiation (IF) because it sacrifices the stability and cohesion of the whole. This exploration promotes implicit learning for all six participants: They can feel palpably the different choices made by each individual either for simultaneous expansion or for inward contraction and conscious body-part control. All participants sense the immediate consequences to movement outcome of their attentional choices and from any microshift in attention.

I have shared this exploration with students as young as 10 years old as they learn initial arabesque skills, and the subtlety of the implicit feedback provides a fascinating self-learning opportunity for more advanced students and even dancers at a professional level. The touch points of the five peers make a lasting imprint that can be used by the dancer or referred to by the teacher at any time in the future. The immediate recall of the sensations of the multidirectional, simultaneous expansion provides a tangible, effective external focus of attention for use in action.

USING TEACHING RESOURCES AS EFFECTIVE EXTERNAL FOCI

Many traditional teaching resources are readily available in some dance studios and provide natural, accessible external foci for all skills levels. Whether it's a hat or a hoop, a ribbon or a scarf, a performance sword or a dagger, stickers, tape, fixed elements such as the barre or the mirror, or more recent technological resources such as mobile phone recording, all can be adapted to harness the EF learning possibilities they provide. The advantages of employing teaching resources are similar to those of using touch – the EF resource promotes not only an immediate effect on learning and improved quality of movement but the lasting impression of dancing with the resource can also be readily recalled later with a simple prompt from the teacher, coach or therapist, which makes for an exceptionally efficient teaching strategy.

USING TEACHING RESOURCES: STICKERS AND TAPE

Stickers and tape can provide an external focus of attention in diverse dance teaching and rehabilitation contexts. For example, during initial skills learning, a star or other inspirational sticker can be used on the breastbone to promote immediate benefits to movement quality and speed in change of direction exercises or to initial turning exercises. The focus might be on 'Where is your star shining?' to correct body orientation, or ask 'How quickly can you shine your star from one corner to the other?' for a cohesive change of direction on diagonal. In the young gymnast study described earlier, a sticker on the breastbone was used to draw the learner's attention to the direction that the sticker points at the end of the turn to enhance the precision of the form in the landing position (Abdollahipour et al. 2014). Stickers are particularly effective with very young dancers: coloured stickers, dots or Mr Smileys can be used on shoes or knees to draw attention to aspects of alignment and to facilitate long-term changes to learning.

In figure 6.8, Emmi is using pink heart stickers instead of partner touch points in a variation of the same balance improvisation described earlier (figure 6.5). The stickers on the back of the hands point down the middle finger, and Emmi takes her attention to the stickers or to the sensation of the stickers and sends energy out from the heart energy centre through the arms in two directions towards the stickers and beyond.

Stability and the reflexive microadjustments necessary for a successful balance are immediately improved through attention to the EF resource. Just as with the partner touch points, stickers are efficient teaching resources because they only need to be used once. The multisensory recall of the sticker (sensation, touch, colour, form) is so vivid that it provides the same benefits as using the real resource and can be referred to at any time by the dancer later whilst dancing. In a rehabilitation context, tape can be used as an EF to draw attention to a desired action to enhance recuperation of movement function or to increase the range of motion. Studies show that by taking the attention to the movement of two pieces of tape on the lower and upper leg, for example, the movement range and the process of rehabilitation of a knee joint can be significantly improved (Wulf 2014).

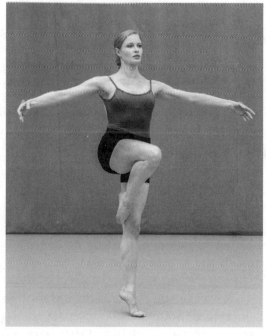

Figure 6.8   Using stickers on the back of the hands as effective external foci. (Emmi)

USING TEACHING RESOURCES: THE BARRE

The ballet barre provides an easy, tangible external focus for students and provides multiple potential attentional functions. Used as a fixed reference point or geometrical line, the barre can enhance understanding of the alignment and the planes of the body (sagittal plane: divides the body in half down the centre line of nose and navel, and movement on this plane is forwards and backwards in parallel to the barre; transverse plane: sections the body horizontally into top and bottom, and movement on this plane is on a level with the barre; coronal plane: divides the body down the centre into front and back, and movement on this plane is towards and away from the barre) or clarify orientation such as en face, ouvert, croisé and écarté or the more subtle line such as epaulement or à dos in relationship to the barre. For certain en l'air positions, the barre provides a fixed 90 degrees from the standing side and a parallel-to-the-floor reference. When a 90-degree leg height is the desired objective the barre provides a fixed point of reference. A 90-degree leg will always be parallel to the barre whether below or above dependent on the height of the dancer. This fixed point of reference also facilitates the visualization of other angles such as 15 degrees for battement glissé or 45 degrees for battement jeté. It can also provide a horizontal reference for the diagonal line of the penché arabesque. Its fixed line gives a point of reference and facilitates orientation in initial quarter and half turns or for actions such as rotation and fouetté.

The barre provides an attentional focus to enhance the quality of transferring weight forwards and backwards (sagittal plane) and gives a sense of the distance travelled as the barre hand slides smoothly with the body. It also helps to orient movements away and towards (coronal plane), measuring the distance travelled and relationship to the barre. Finally, the students' attention can be taken to the quality of their touch on the barre. They can feel the sensation of the wood as they slide along the barre in a transfer-of-weight action. They can also use it as an imaginary partner dancer, focusing on the use of appropriate touch, such as lightness or a firm press downwards as used in partnering, to promote the desired upper back support (rather than common barre actions of gripping or pulling upwards that increase counterproductive tension and distort the line).

Traditional ballet class is organized in such a way that learning at the barre and in the centre is typically an isolating experience: Students are at best focusing on the back of the head of the student in front or at worst, straight into a wall or the mirror. This isolation exacerbates our human tendency for self-related thought and body-part adjustment. A simple but effective modification is to pair students so that barre exercises are done facing or mirroring one another (figure 6.9). This provides immediate benefits because dancers focus on the same movements (movement effect) done by a partner dancer, which creates a natural external focus for learning. This teaching strategy can function on multiple levels:

- The students can aim to mirror the movements and the quality of one another and to focus on their relationship and the dancing space between them. Their attention to the movement outcome and quality are thereby heightened throughout the exercise.

- Students immediately engage socially and smile, learning feels lighter, and motivation for learning is enhanced. The dancer's focus is taken far from the self-related thought of isolated learning.

- The benefits promoted by the external focus mean that technical aspects of the exercise are immediately improved for *both* students. These include aspects such as strength, balance, precision, speed and stamina.

- Students of different skills levels or with different qualities can be paired so that their learning is complemented.

- Speed of learning is improved and learning is more readily embodied. This leads to long-term changes in the learning experienced.

Just as happens when using the other teaching resources as an EF, the impressions created at the barre can be recalled later when practicing in the centre. This includes the lasting impression of the fixed presence of the barre, the experience of sociably sharing exercises and the presence and mirror image of a barre partner.

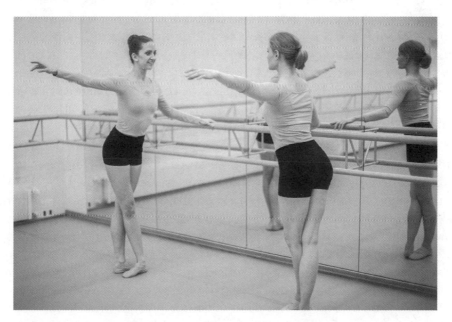

Figure 6.9   A barre partner provides multilevel EF advantages. (Kailey and Emmi)

USING TEACHING RESOURCES: THE MIRROR AND VISUAL RECORDINGS

Teachers in my workshops frequently ask whether the use of the mirror in dance promotes an external or an internal focus. They have similar questions about the extensive referencing of video and visual recordings by young dancers today on social media.

The role of the mirror in attentional focus is a logical question because the mirror is clearly an external resource and yet, without guided use, it can draw our attention precisely to amplify the focus on the self. The answer is that the mirror in and of itself is neither EF nor IF. The attentional focus depends entirely on *how* we choose to use it and the way we instruct students to use the mirror as a resource. If we guide students to attend to the height of the *leg* in the mirror or to look where their *shoulders* are, then we as teachers are clearly instructing them to use the mirror to intensify the focus on conscious, self-related control (IF). Equally, if we give no guidance at all on the appropriate use of the mirror as a resource, we expose students to the natural human inclination to reflect on aspects of the physical self. We could alternatively instruct students to use the mirror to reach for a true diagonal line, to self-check that their jump is vertical, or to check their spacing in relation to other dancers. In this way, we are promoting an external focus of attention and teaching an appropriate use of the mirror as a learning resource.

Video and mobile phone recording for student feedback can provide excellent EF resources that dancers of today's generation can particularly relate to because this is a medium they are comfortable with. Results depend on the *how* – how we choose to guide the attention of students and dancers whilst using recordings as a teaching resource. If it's a video of another inspirational artist that students might watch on YouTube, then take this as an opportunity to draw their attention to EF elements such as the line of a movement, the flow, a quality or dynamic, the musicality of a particular step or perhaps the artist's dramatic interpretation or charismatic communication with the audience. For consolidated interactive learning, ask the students to identify the elements that make this an exceptional performance. In my experience, students' responses are surprising. Even students as young as 12 years old will spontaneously identify all those EF elements. Rarely do they respond that it's the height of the leg, the point of the foot or the angle of the back that make this performance outstanding, even if these are precisely the body-part elements they obsess over when left without teacher viewing guidance.

Filming individual or group exercises is quick and easy to do and, when the dancer's attention is guided, provides an excellent, effective teaching opportunity, even between exercises, to develop student self-feedback and goal-setting abilities. It's a natural human tendency that when left to our own devices watching a film of our performance without attentional guidance, we focus on our body parts or on our own perceived faults and defects, the same as we do with the mirror. This tendency is known to be heightened when the activity is physical movement and is a public activity (Wulf 2013). When sharing film with a dancer or student, therefore, I guide them by asking them first to identify three aspects of their performance that they liked or felt were good and we name those elements 'keepers', the three foundational elements that they would like to maintain in the future. Then I ask them to identify their wish list of one to three desired elements they would like to propose as their next goals to build upon their established keepers. They might, for example, identify goals such as to find more speed in a certain section, to focus on stability in a movement by pressing down or to increase the extension line or the suspension. The number of goals depends on their skill level and maturity. This might be just one wish on the list for younger students, but three is a manageable, measurable, achievable target for more advanced students and professionals. Less is more with goals, too, to promote selective successful, embedded learning and optimal attention and focus. Build the goals on the performance wish list like building blocks little by little, being sure to reinforce and maintain the foundational blocks, the keepers, every time.

I'm always surprised by how accurate the students' observations are. If I can be quiet and resist the temptation to impose the goal, students frequently identify precisely the next priorities I would have wished. Permitting students to set their own goals brings many further learning and performance enhancement benefits that we will explore in chapter 7, increasing responsibility and ownership for learning and promoting intrinsic motivation.

USING IMAGERY AS AN EFFECTIVE EXTERNAL FOCUS

Imagery for dance is defined as 'a consciously created mental representation of an experience either real or imaginary that may affect the dancer and her or his movement' (Pavlik and Nordin-Bates 2016, 51). The use of imagery is natural to the creative process, to the sharing of choreographic material and to individual artistic interpretation. In dance training and performance, we already regularly employ imagery, particularly metaphorical imagery, and we are seemingly creative with the content and the extent of the implementation in comparison to other movement disciplines (Pavlik and Nordin-Bates 2016; Guss-West and Wulf 2016). Just as happens with the use of touch, dance teachers tend to use imagery spontaneously in class and not necessarily as part of a systematic teaching strategy. Research suggests that teaching would be more effective if imagery choice was planned together with the preparation of learning outcomes and lesson plans, with a systematic planning of how to implement it throughout the class. Imagery should be appropriate to the learning outcomes or rehearsal objectives then, and to the particular dance context, student group or dancing public. Studies indicate that the imagery used needs to be relevant and personalized for the imager or student. The imager's or student's preferences, learning styles and feelings should be taken into consideration, otherwise the effectiveness of an imagery-based EF teaching strategy is undermined (Pavlik and Nordin-Bates 2016).

Findings also suggest that the ability to use imagery needs to be taught in parallel with the student's technical development (Pavlik and Nordin-Bates 2016). You may have noticed in your own teaching practice that not all students have the same ability to image visually, to 'see' a movement in the mind or mind's eye, or to image kinaesthetically, to imagine the 'feel' of the movement effectively. There also appear to be differences in the ability to effectively integrate and embody that imagery so that it informs the physical movement quality, energy, dynamics and appropriate tension. In Western dance class, time is not typically set aside to develop attention and imaging skills as it is in Eastern movement practice where attention and focus constitute one of the three foundations for successful movement and are developed in parallel with the foundation of posture and alignment (figure 3.1). Performance psychologist Dr Sanna Nordin-Bates suggests that even if dance teachers plan to introduce imagery ability training into class, given the pressure on teachers to achieve certain levels of physical technique, this additional training might at best amount to five minutes of class time, which falls far short of recommendations in high-level sports (Pavlik and Nordin-Bates 2016).

In research studies participants who had the most developed imagery abilities tended to be those with a preference for a kinaesthetic learning style, those who preferred learning through feeling and practical experiencing. However, studies suggest that all dancers can increase their imagery ability and conclude that these skills can be learnt (Pavlik and Nordin-Bates 2016).

One of the strategies we might use to develop this ability is to choose a theme for appropriate imagery when planning class. When we use imagery extensively in class, the danced experience of those images can feel like a string of consecutive diverse foci: one for this action, another for the next step and so on. Dancers do their best to find the logic or find associations between the images to facilitate the flow of the dance, as if dancing a series of film images. This can be challenging if the teaching images are arbitrary and unrelated to each other. Dancers might receive such diverse teaching imagery as whipped like a cappuccino, be a shooting star and push down against a rubber swimming ring, all within one movement phrase. Choosing a theme for the imagery while planning a class – for example, a water, energy, winter or at the beach theme, depending on the level and the nature of the specific learning group – facilitates dancers' attentional focus, enabling them to consolidation the imagery and create a kind of logic dancing road map or coherent film. Dancers can more adeptly imagine when imagery is themed or grouped and, therefore, immerse themselves deeper in the details of the imagery, rendering the use of imagery more effective (Nordin-Bates 2019). Theming imagery also stimulates our creativity as a teacher. I have developed surprising and effective class imagery that I would never have otherwise thought of by imposing a creative theme on myself that was appropriate for the students. This is particularly effective when facilitating learning and developing imagery ability for older adult dancers and dancing publics with special needs and challenges.

Attention and Focus in Practice

GUIDING MULTISENSORY IMAGERY

Dr Sanna Nordin-Bates, senior lecturer in sport and dance psychology

Most people understand that imagery, artistry and storytelling are an inherent part of children's dance, and almost everyone knows that's what professional dancers do: embody a story. In the middle, it can get lost completely. If the imagery of you *loving that person* or *picking this flower* is serious enough and worthy of a professional performance, then why isn't it good enough in the studio?

Using imagery needs guidance at first to support a mindful 'learning to observe'. It's not just 'flow like a fountain'; it's also 'Where is that sensation of water?', 'How high is it going?', 'Feel that right at the top'. Usually we don't go into so much detail. A Dance for Parkinson's Disease teacher shared that she found 'Reach up to pick the apple' effective; however, if she added 'Where is the tree?', 'Is it associated with a nice memory?', 'What colour is the apple?', the image would become multisensory and stimulate attention better. You wouldn't do that every time because it takes too long and maybe not everybody liked it. Eventually, the image becomes embodied and you could perhaps just say 'fountain' because they've worked on it and that very basic descriptive image is effective.

In terms of stages of learning, with automaticity comes cognitive space and freedom. What are you going to do with that cognitive space? The risk is you'll either start thinking about technical details that should be automatic, about toast or about what to do on Saturday. Dancers don't often have an alternative go-to focus when the original image is no longer necessary or no longer engaging. The movement becomes habitual. You need to keep it fresh, and that's when characterization or musicality or other creative attentional foci can really come in. If it's more conscious control, comparison, mirrors and critique, of course, it's not going to be engaging and immersing. It will only really work if you are able to step into the story.

Any metaphorical image that we might choose has the potential to promote an external focus of attention that will draw the attention to the movement objective or effect and away from the conscious adjustment of body parts. However, imagery like many of the other potential EF types (figure 2.3) is in and of itself neither EF nor IF. *How* we direct the dancer's attention and *how* we word our instructions and cues are what assure that the image will promote an external attentional focus enabling optimal learning and performance outcome. It is not the imagery content itself. So it's not the fact that I chose a fountain, to stay with the same analogy, that makes it an effective EF, but *how* I choose to draw dancers' attention to the potential qualities or sensory information inherent in that image. It's completely possible to instruct using metaphorical imagery and inadvertently direct the focus back onto the self. For example, when working with the shoulder blades, I might say 'Imagine the flat sliding action like a wing that draws in and down' (EF) and then follow up with 'Try to move your shoulders in this way' (IF). This teaching instruction begins with a metaphorical image and ends with an instruction that brings attention back to a body-part control that would counteract any benefits promoted by use of the imagery. As an alternative, we could have identified the action first by sensing the movement in a floor exercise or focusing the attention on the movement in a peer touch exercise and then added metaphorical imagery to consolidate the learning with no mention of the body part itself at all.

As an alternative movement imagery, using what is termed *direct imagery*, *mental rehearsal* or *3D visualization* of one's own optimal movement pathway through space can be used in place of actually physically marking an exercise. This promotes all the benefits of an external focus: movement efficiency, speed, fluidity and precision. This is the type of imagery most used in sport training and yet we don't employ it so often in dance.

> Mental imagery impacts many cognitive processes in the brain: motor control, attention, perception, planning, and memory. So the brain is getting trained for actual performance during visualization. (Adams 2009, para. 5)

Every time we physically execute a new movement, we are laying down the neural pathway and recording holographic, proprioceptive information along the way. The more we repeat a potentially unhelpful pattern whilst we mark movements – incorrect coordination, uneconomic engagement of resources or inappropriate tension – the more we embed them. Incorrect proprioceptive learning or an imprecise movement pathway must then be unlearnt and rerecorded in order to eventually master the movement. In this sense, it is more effective to first visualize, for example, the perfect dynamic balance and rhythm of a triple pirouette or the ideal movement trajectory and the proprioceptive feeling or the breath of the grand jeté en tournant. Physical marking can be easily substituted in class by a rapid, closed-eye visualization of the ideal movement outcome before executing an exercise. In my own direct experience, even with young students, this results in less incorrect repetition during initial skills learning and less need for basic teacher feedback on the movement form.

> . . . researchers . . . have investigated brain activation patterns during visual (what a movement looks like) and kinetic (*kinesthetic*) imagery (what a movement feels like). All found that kinetic imagery closely resembles execution by activating motor preparation, refining motor abilities, and initiating supportive physiological changes. (Karin and Nordin-Bates 2019, 2)

A TEACHER'S EXTERNAL FOCUS OF ATTENTION

Teaching with an external attentional focus approach as our chosen movement control strategy, as we have seen, concerns initially *how* we choose to word our teaching instructions and cues for optimum learning and enhanced movement outcomes of our students; however, external focus theory can also be considered from a much broader perspective. When we reflect, we begin to appreciate that we can also adopt an external focus ourselves in relation to our own teaching practice, to promote personal mental, physical and energy benefits. Rather than focusing on the self – How am *I* teaching this lesson? I wonder what they are thinking about *my* teaching? – we might shift our attention away from the self to focus on the *effect* of our teaching. We could, for example, shift to How are *they* experiencing the class? How are *they* receiving this information?

An external attentional focus approach can be applied to enhance the outcome of any activity in any work context. Actor Bill Irwin, for example, during an interview on *NPR Weekend Edition*, spoke about the same phenomenon, the relationship of successful acting to external focus.

> . . . most important for an actor, the responsibility is who am I speaking to, so when you go into the "Sesame Street" studio . . . you have to think about the kids and their parents who are watching and what is the kernel of story that needs to be told. . . . Let what you want or what the character wants guide you. Otherwise you're thinking about – am I good? Should I be loud enough? Am I handsome here? And then you're dead. (Lyden 2009, para. 41-42)

When Irwin takes his attention to the audience, to the essence of the story or what the character wants he is acting using a consistent external focus of attention. As soon as he shifts his attentional focus back to 'am I good?',

TABLE 6.1   Examples of External Focus Types to Address Different Learning Styles

EF TYPE	LEARNING STYLE	EXAMPLES OF APPLICATION
Teacher, peer demonstration	Multimodal	A demonstration of the global movement: form, quality, dynamics, energy, appropriate effort, breath, intention, attention and focus
Tangible, physical object	Multimodal	Press the floor, push down on the barre, stretch your tights, reach into your shoes, fill your leotard, lift up through your zip line, push up into your hat
Resources	Visual	A picture or drawing of the movement form or effect, a picture or drawing of a metaphoric image to promote the desired form or quality
	Kinaesthetic	A video of an artist executing an exemplary movement form, quality or dynamic; a video of a dancer's own movement
Artistic focus cues	Multimodal	Focus on the drama, on the emotion, on the prop; work with your costume; focus on your partner dancer, on the relationship; focus on the rhythm, on the music, on the text, on a particular instrument, on the singer, on the breathing of the singer or instrumentalist, on the space between you and your partner; focus on communicating with the audience
Sounds, sounding and voice	Auditory	Hear the quality of the landing, hear the frappé or strike, hear the glissé, the chassé, the swoosh; hear your out-breath; hear the rhythm of the tapping, the attack of the zapateado, the quality of clapping, the sounding of the teacher
Directional focus cues	Visual	Long, short, straight, out, in, up, open, closed, crossed, diagonal, zigzag, curvy, wavy, small, big, fold, bend, crease, straighten, push, press, reach, stretch, rotate
Qualitative focus cues	Kinaesthetic	Smooth, sharp, accent, dab, shoot, strike, quick, whip, flick, powerful, melting, radiating, fluid, delicate, contract, expand, make space, allow, elongate, suspend, heavy, falling, rebound, resist
Geometrical focus cues	Visual	Circle, triangle, square, angle, straight line, spiral, figure-8, en croix (in a cross), diagonal, horizontal, vertical, parallel, 3D, hologram, five lines in space
French ballet vocabulary	Multimodal	Plié, tendu, glissé, developpé, fondu, frappé, coupé, battement, ballotté, arabesque, balancé, pas de chat, renversé, en dehors, en dedans, rotation, fouetté
Proprioceptive	Kinaesthetic	Feel the pressure, feel the contrast, feel the strike, feel the spiral, feel flat, feel the twist, feel the warmth, feel the touch, feel the opening, make space, allow energy to flow
Metaphoric imagery	Kinaesthetic	Like honey, push through water, like sticky chewing gum, move through grass, like chopping a cucumber, on hot sand, push the sand, embrace something, gather champagne energy
	Visual	Spiraling like a tornado, unfolding like a leaf, like a shooting star, powerful centre like a geyser, expanding like the sun, reach for the stars, like a cat, add colours

'am I loud enough?' and 'am I handsome?' he is working with an IF and in his words, then he's 'dead'!

Similarly, writer Marianne Williamson shares that the key for a writer is also to have a focus beyond the self. When she begins her working day, if her focus is on herself or on maintaining her own best-seller status (IF), then her thoughts are fragmented and her focus is limited, she observes; whereas when she begins with the thought that her writing would be of service to others (EF), she finds, 'my nervous system responds with a sense of focus and clarity I do not otherwise have. My mind opens vibrantly to its natural talents' (Williamson 2004, 118).

Bringing our attention to the process of our attention is a lifelong process. Although scientific research might infer logically that integrating an EF movement control approach 100 per cent of the time would be the optimal goal, life and art are rarely polarized in such a way. Start to notice when and why you draw students' attention to the conscious control of their body parts, in

---

Attention and Focus in Practice

ENHANCING TECHNIQUE AND ARTISTRY SIMULTANEOUSLY

Raymond Chai, teacher, ballet master, choreographer, former professional dancer

Both internal and external focus of attention are control strategies. It's perhaps just easier as a teacher to unthinkingly use internal focus in a command style, as we feel as if we are being more tangible for students, more effective. However, the student is passive with this control approach and becomes dependent on the constant physical feedback of the teacher (encouraging explicit learning). Using an external focus provides tools for the dancer and induces their engagement in their own learning (encouraging implicit learning). The student must experiment to begin to know and eventually master their *own* body. Since I've been teaching and choreographing, I see the importance of embracing this approach, and it's so much easier if we start using it from the beginning of our training! I believe that dancers (and teachers) today should try to attain this shift. I think it's important as so many teachers try *not* to use the word technique, as if it hinders artistry and kills the 'dance', when they are actually so intertwined. When you adopt an external focus, you enhance all simultaneously: power, precision and artistry. You never have to negate the importance or the necessity of technique for the sake of artistry.

what teaching contexts. When under pressure, for example, it's only natural that we reach for our habitual, most accessible neural pathways and revert back to teach in a way that is deeply embedded or in which we ourselves learnt. Aim simply at first to develop consciousness of the impact of shifting attention and then perhaps approach the introduction of external focus more as a sliding scale. Ask yourself, How much of the time am I already promoting an external focus of attention in my teaching? How and when could I easily choose to use EF more often?

In other movement learning contexts, such as sport and physiotherapy, we know that teachers, coaches and therapists without attentional focus training do promote an external focus of attention some of the time (10 to 20 per cent) (Porter, Wu and Partridge 2010). In dance practice, we know that we use an external focus more than in a sports context as we frequently use metaphorical imagery, and some teachers may also use traditional ballet vocabulary, so we are probably already promoting an external focus of attention in our classes 20 to 50 per cent of our teaching time without consciously choosing to make a change. Any increase in the time spent promoting an EF that we can introduce will provide immediate benefits to the effectiveness of our teaching and to our student's capacity to learn and will also provide improvements to dancers' performance outcome.

Set a realistic goal for yourself at first that you believe you can achieve. As suggested in chapter 2, aim to promote external focus for about 50 per cent of your teaching time or therapy practice instructions at first. After 10 years of teaching with awareness of my attentional focus choices, working with diverse populations that include professional dancers, teachers, older adult dancers and therapists, my usage ratio of EF to IF still varies depending on the context. On a good day while teaching live class in the studio, with a group of students or dancers I know, I manage to use an EF control approach about 90 per cent of the time. When I do use a teaching instruction that draws students' attention back onto the conscious control of a body part rather than onto the desired effect of their movements, a metaphorical buzzer goes off in my head, and I smile to myself and make a mental note. I reflect an instant and ask myself, Could I have done that differently? Can I do that differently next time?

REFLECTION PROMPTS

- Has Western dance teaching always displayed a predominance of IF control approach? Find examples on the Internet of inspirational or older-generation teachers that you admire and listen and observe for a moment their chosen teaching control approach. What is their priority focus in their feedback and cueing? How much of the time are they promoting a focus onto the control of a body part (IF)? Or are they naturally focusing more on the desired effect, quality or outcome of the movement (EF)? If they are using predominantly EF, how are they doing that? See whether you can identify and jot down a few external focus types that they are perhaps using intuitively (refer to figure 2.3).

- It presents a metacognitive attentional challenge to teach class and also observe yourself teaching at the same time! An effective resource for supporting this attentional development is to film or record a class for later viewing. Observing yourself teaching with a little 'distance' provides a much clearer picture of what your habitual control choices are. As with the inspirational teacher films, try first to identify two or three examples of when you spontaneously use an external focus in your instructions and feedback. Can you identify the types of EF you already use (figure 2.3)? Do you notice a pattern? When do you typically use EF? Is it related to the skill level of the dancers? Or is it related to the particular movement task? The dance style or perhaps the context (e.g., exam preparation versus free choreography)?

- It's a good idea to brainstorm a list in your inspirational journal of your own favourite EF 'ingredients'. Reflect on some of the areas we have explored:

  - The types of EF foci that you already like to use
  - Descriptive, qualitative or geometric EF vocabulary that you already use that works for your dance context
  - The touch points that you have used that were effective or some that you would like to introduce that seem appropriate for your dance context or students
  - Imagery themes that you might try

- Review and adjust your list regularly at first to refine what works and what doesn't work so well. You can refer to your brainstorm ingredient list whilst *cooking up* your lesson plans or keep it close to hand as a prompt in class to stimulate your creativity as you go along.

CHAPTER 7

BEYOND ATTENTIONAL FOCUS

. . . learning is not simply a function of the task information provided to the learner . . . it is subject to a variety of social-cognitive-affective influences that may also, intentionally or unintentionally, be conveyed.

Gabriele Wulf (in Wulf et al. 2010, 1)

As we develop our consciousness of the process of attention and we become aware of *how* we are cueing our own attention in dance or how we are directing dancers' attention when we are teaching, it's perhaps pertinent to put attentional focus into a broader movement learning context. Attentional focus is one foundational element in a broader theory of movement learning that, when combined with other motivational strategies, brings further incremental physical and mental benefits to learning and performance. This holistic combination of mindful attentional focus and motivational strategies identifies the respect and *autonomy* of the individual as central to increased intrinsic motivation and, therefore, optimal performance (Wulf and Lewthwaite 2016).

Supporting the autonomy of the dancer has not typically been a priority in many professional Western dance institutions in the last decades, and yet research shows that a training approach and environment that support the autonomy of the performer are precisely the conditions necessary to enable excellence in physical and mental performance.

The OPTIMAL (optimizing performance through intrinsic motivation and attention for learning) theory of motor learning (Wulf and Lewthwaite 2016) is made up of three main elements, one attentional and two motivational: the systematic implementation of an **external focus of attention** in training, which we have already explored, plus two motivational strategies referred to as **autonomy support** and **enhanced expectancy** (Lewthwaite et al. 2015). This combination is shown to facilitate fluency in brain–body systems functioning in a virtuous circle, such that when the elements are continually implemented as part of a coaching and teaching strategy, each one increases the beneficial effect of the next to further promote optimal movement and learning in a cycle of continual improvement (Wulf et al. 2018). Research provides exciting evidence of this combination as an effective and efficient, holistic, high-performance training approach. Supporting the autonomy of the performer is not only a desirable training 'soft skill', but findings show that the cumulative effect of adopting these holistic elements also produces 'hard facts', or performance enhancements, such as increased maximum power or force production, jump height, speed and precision. These findings apply to all skill levels and occur throughout diverse movement learning contexts, including rehabilitation and recovery. This combination approach not only has the potential to affect movement skills learning and outcome but also can be used in a broader context to enhance complementary skills such as communication and listening.

One of the first elements to consider when choosing to support the autonomy of the performer is our use of teaching, or self-cueing, **language**. Do we use a controlling language or one that gives freedom and space to the individual? Do we select vocabulary that *enables* movement and high performance or that inadvertently *disables* performance? What tone do we use with ourselves in self-talk and inner dialogue?

The deliberate introduction of an element of **choice** into training and learning is another strategy to support a sense of autonomy; even seemingly inconsequential choices are shown to promote a higher performance outcome. Choice as a strategy in dance training might range from inconsequential choices such as 'Would you like to start that to the left or to the right?' to giving dancers the choice for more responsibility for their own learning, even to quite young students, or introducing freedom of choice for learners to set their own goal. The other element of the theory involves consciously **enhancing learner expectancy** and aiming to mitigate perceived difficulty. These elements all contribute incrementally to further enhance movement outcome.

Let's take a brief look at these motivational elements and their potential application – at why we might want to consider them alongside developing attentional focus awareness in dance. And, how can they be translated for dance training and implemented into a day-to-day class or rehearsal context?

SUPPORTING THE AUTONOMY OF THE DANCER

Having the ability to control our own actions, or being **autonomous**, is defined as a basic human psychological need (Deci and Ryan 2000), and research shows that people are prepared to make more effort and work harder for an option that leads to a choice (Wulf and Lewthwaite 2016).

Supporting an individual's need for autonomy brings multifaceted benefits such as promoting self-regulation, enhancing motivation for learning and a more active involvement in their own learning, which leads to a deeper processing of information. It's relatively well established in motor learning research that motivation, learning and performance are improved when learners have some degree of control over their own environment and their own actions. Supporting autonomy in a movement learning context might include giving performers the ability to make decisions about their training conditions and the amount of practice they need, and some influence over when and how they receive skills demonstration and feedback, for example (Wulf and Lewthwaite 2016).

The traditional, Western dance teaching style, known as command style (Mosston and Ashworth 1994), is a teacher-centric style in which the voice of the learner is seldom and in some cases never encouraged. It is an approach that can still be seen today as part of the 'received wisdom' of teaching handed down through generations. This teaching style, however, is unnecessarily restrictive and controlling of learners, their learning process and their learning environment. Research suggests that performers in a controlling environment have additionally to suppress negative emotional reactions due to their lack of choice or influence over outcomes and that this undermines their ability to remain focused on the movement task (Reeve and Tseng 2011). A controlling teaching style is ineffective and counterproductive to the pursuit of high performance standards. When taken to an extreme, as witnessed in certain dance contexts, it is uncreative and can be damaging for the art according to Christopher Hampson, artistic director of Scottish Ballet, who suggests that 'those that consistently shout at people or deprive them of guidance to gain respect should know this is the "fools" way. It may deliver a short burst of focus to some dancers, but it evaporates shortly thereafter' (Hampson 2018). The desire for exactitude, precision and movement correctness could be more effectively achieved through supportive language and by implementing simple elements of choice that enable the dancer to have a sense of autonomy and control over outcomes.

SUPPORTING AUTONOMY – LANGUAGE

The social–cognitive–affective influences on movement skills learning are perhaps most easily observed when we begin to consider the impact of our choice of instructional language. For the sake of research, instructional language is divided into two generalized polarities: wording that allows the learner a sense of choice and autonomy (autonomy-supportive language) versus language that aims to control and allows few options for an individual approach to training or mastering a movement (controlling language).

In a research study measuring precision and accuracy in motor skills learning (a bowling action), participants were divided into three groups. The first group received learning instructions in controlling language, and the second group received instructions in autonomy-supportive language (table 7.1). The third group received instructions in as neutral a language as possible to act as a research control group (Hooyman, Wulf and Lewthwaite 2014).

TABLE 7.1   Controlling Versus Supportive Language

CONTROLLING LANGUAGE	SUPPORTIVE LANGUAGE
Today you will learn _____ and perform it well.	Today is your opportunity to learn _____.
You may not begin until you are told to do so.	Please wait until the instruction has ended to begin.
Make sure all of the elements are organized in their respective places. You may only use one at a time.	You may organize the elements in any way you prefer.
You must maintain a consistent pace.	Feel free to go at a pace you are comfortable with.
When initiating _____, you must take the movement directly over the shoulder. Do not take it out to the side.	Here is a hint for achieving your best _____. When starting, you may want to take the movement vertically.

Based on Hooyman, Wulf and Lewthwaite (2014).

The impact of the instructional language on immediate performance and also on longer-term learning was measured. Long-term learning was assessed by measuring the performance several days later in trials in which no further instructions were given. The open, friendly language of the supportive column of table 7.1 that gave a sense of freedom from controlling restraints and room for individuality and offered hints for how to master the technique rather than commands consistently promoted an increased speed of mastery and performance precision. This difference was maintained when the exercise was revisited several days after receiving initial instructions, indicating improved learning retention with supportive instruction language. Allowing learners some degree of autonomy appears to enhance their confidence in their ability and minimize the need to manage negative emotional responses. Autonomy support appears to promote pleasant feelings or positive emotions that are thought to enable consolidation of movement recall (Hooyman, Wulf and Lewthwaite 2014).

In practice, the choice of teaching language might not be such a black or white, controlling versus supportive scenario as the research described. Teachers and coaches probably use more of a sliding scale of controlling language versus autonomy-supportive language and this choice of language might shift depending on the particular dancers, student group, learning context or their mood. This is not a question just for teachers and coaches, however. Bringing our attention to our choice of language doesn't concern only the language we use in public, it also requires us to become aware of the language we use intimately with ourselves in self-talk and self-cueing. Our own mindset and the instructional language we choose to use with ourselves can be our own worst enemy in terms of achieving our best performance. For some dancers and teachers, it's our own inner voice that uses ferociously controlling and unsupportive language. (See exploration 5.5 for more on developing awareness of self-talk and inner dialogue.)

Once we start to become conscious of the power of our choice of teaching and self-cueing language, it's interesting to reflect on the actual words that we typically use in individual movement instruction. Are the words we use adapted to the task? Are they particularly effective? Or do we adopt them unconsciously? Listening to dance teachers teach all over the world, I hear wonderful, creative variations from those who have consciously chosen to reflect on the impact of their instructional language. However, I also frequently hear the same, limited instructional vocabulary whatever the language or skill levels: stay, hold, squeeze, grip, pull up, turn out, bend, contract, stop. Here is a professional level instruction for concluding a pirouette, for example: 'Hold the position a little bit more—gluteus in and up, turn out the standing leg, open the knee and stay!' (Boesch 2018).

Until we become aware of our habitual choices and decide to consciously experiment with the effect of different teaching and cueing vocabulary, we will tend to use, for the most part unconsciously, the vocabulary that we were taught in and have always heard. Let's explore the difference in the effect of a few instruction words so that you can feel the immediate response of your own body. This exploration compares hold versus sustain, pull up versus extend, and turn out versus spiral. However, you can easily substitute these for another two words of your choice that you feel give similar instructional information.

EXPLORATION 7.1 – THE EFFECT OF DIFFERENT INSTRUCTION WORDS

Find a space and take a position of your choice for an easy balance on one foot, either flat foot or demi-pointe. It could be a low arabesque, a balance on one foot with the other sur le cou-de-pied or parallel retiré, for example. Let's start with the words **hold** and **sustain**.

Take up your balance position and start to instruct yourself out loud or in your head by repeating the word **hold** as if you were marking a slow musical bar: and **hold**, two, three, four . . . **hold** . . . **hold** . . . **hold**. Notice, if you can, the sensations in your body of tension or effort or lightness and ease. Observe your breathing. Continuing with your balance position, change the rhythmic instruction word to **sustain**: and **sustain**, two, three, four . . . **sustain** . . . **sustain** . . . **sustain**.

Did you notice anything happen in your body when you changed the word? Was your muscle tension the same with each word? How was your breathing with each word? How big did the movement feel with each word?

Let's look now at the difference between **pull up** and **extend** using a position or balance on two feet of your choice. This might be in parallel, in natural or classical first, fourth or fifth position or other, flat foot or demi-pointe with arms of your choice. Instruct yourself repeatedly to **pull up**: and **pull up**, two, three, four . . . **pull up** . . . **pull up** . . . and **pull up**. Observe your body and its sensations. And come down and shake out if you need to. Continue with the same two-foot balance, but change the instruction word to **extend**: and **extend**, two, three, four . . . **extend** . . . **extend** . . . and **extend**.

What did you notice as you performed your balance? Was the balance more successful with one word or the other? Did anything about the quality of the balance change when you changed words? Was one balance more spacious or freer than the other, for example?

And let's take our last example, the difference between **turn out** and **spiral**. Stand on both feet in a classical first or fifth position or extend a 'playing' leg in a pointed dégagé position and instruct yourself insistently as if on a rhythmic pulse to **turn out**: and **turn out**, two, three, four . . . **turn out** . . . **turn out** . . . and **turn out**. Scan the body for sensations. And, continue by changing the word to **spiral**: and **spiral**, two, three, four . . . **spiral** . . . **spiral** . . . **spiral**.

How did your body change when the word changed? Did your whole posture change? Was the effort different with a different word? Where was your focus with each word: inwards towards the body movement (IF) or outwards in the direction of the movement (EF)? Which felt easier or more pleasurable?

Jot down your immediate observations – the physical or sensory changes that occurred as the word changed or emotions, colours, energy or images that were prompted by the different words – for your later reference. Answer spontaneously without analyzing which words gave you a sense of dance and a sense of freedom.

A word in and of itself is a neutral vessel. It's a sound and could carry any meaning. Words become coloured by meaning through our collective agreement of their meaning. Different words convey different energetic intentions. Meaning is open to interpretation and varies from language to language, and individuals might have their own nuanced, visceral or proprioceptive understanding of the energetic intention of a word. Nevertheless, some generalizations can be made regarding the impact of the choice of instructional words on physical outcome and the quality of performance. Once you start to explore, you will sense that some instructional words seem to convey an energetic intention that blocks the natural outward flow of the movement or perhaps restricts the expansion of the breath. Some words seem to convey a sense of space for movement and a sense of freedom and flow, whilst others provoke a feeling of limitation or imply a rigid finite action that arrives and stops, even when, at face value, the two words might appear to describe the same basic action. Developing our awareness of the choice of our words and their power to enable or disable movement enhances enormously our teaching effectiveness.

Table 7.2 lists words that we frequently hear in dance training that have the potential to disable optimum movement. They imply a finite movement with a fixed end point or a stopped or held position. They encourage the use of inappropriate amounts of effort and suboptimal breathing and can reinforce a focus inwards onto body-part control (IF). You probably can think of many more words that disturb your dancing when you hear them! As we saw when exploring an Eastern approach to movement and the nature of universal energy in our movements, there is no such thing as 'hold' or 'stay' and no such thing as 'stop'. An energy molecule cannot stop, so there is no human possibility to hold a balance or fix a pirouette position. To harness the nature of energy flow and to promote successful reflexive movement, we need to enable the continuity of the flow rather than inadvertently restrict it by our choice of words.

In the second column of table 7.2 are alternative words to support a sense of movement continuity, give a sense of space for the individual and a focus on the effect of the movement and thus enable physical performance. These suggestions are far from exhaustive but are a starting point for brainstorming creative alternatives to promote a particular desired effect.

The third column is what is termed grammatically the **gerund**. In the gerund form, the word is no longer a **verb**. It's not something you have to do and is no longer an instruction. It is a **noun**. This grammatical construction does not exist in every language. However, if you have the possibility, introduce it rather than the verb instruction into your teaching or self-cueing wherever you can. In my experience, it further enhances the dancer's sense of infinite continuity, possibility and external focus. The gerund is free of subject and object, of you and me. It is free of the self and the body part and is just something to be experienced. If I give you the instruction 'extend' (action verb), for example, it's me instructing you. Even though it would be an external focus instruction, it still implies that *your* leg should extend. Whereas if I simply say 'and extending', there is no you, no subject, only sharing, sensing and extending. Using the gerund form offers a greater abstraction and sense of freedom to focus the attention further from the self and onto the extending effect of the movement. When we take the 'I' out of it, there is no separation, no 'I' that dances, only dancing and oneness.

The recognition of the social–cognitive–affective influences on movement skills learning and performance outcome acknowledges that effective teaching involves this kind of holistic, multidimensional reflection and awareness. Finnish teacher Timo Kokkonen reminds us that meaning goes beyond even the choice of a word and that ultimately 'intention is everything!' He suggests that sometimes in dance what might seem like negative or controlling words on paper can 'pass' and have a motivational effect *if* the teacher's intention is supportive and loving (Kokkonen 2019). The opposite is also true. Many of us have been the target of sugary, 'loving' words delivered with a wounding intention, like a poisoned dart, that have undermined our ability to perform.

TABLE 7.2   Potentially Disabling Instruction Words and Enabling Alternatives

DISABLING	ENABLING	GERUND
Stay	Flow, float, suspend, fly, glide, surf, enjoy	Flowing, floating, suspending, flying, gliding, surfing, enjoying
Hold	Sustain, grow, expand, smile	Sustaining, growing, expanding, smiling
Squeeze	Spiral, press, twist	Spiraling, pressing, twisting
Grip	Encircle, maintain, sustain	Encircling, maintaining, sustaining
Pull up	Lengthen, elongate, extend	Lengthening, elongating, extending
Turn out	Rotate, spiral, open	Rotating, spiraling, opening
Bend	Reach, curve, arc, fold, melt, soften, hang	Reaching, curving, arcing, folding, melting, softening, hanging
Contract	Resist, push, round	Resisting, pushing, rounding
Stop	Close, descend, conclude, diminish, return	Closing, descending, concluding, diminishing, returning

Take any word as an example, such as the word *sorry*. It's complex and multidimensional, and there must be myriad interpretations of what that word might mean in practice. Almost no two people have exactly the same nuanced understanding. Now apply that same thinking to a movement instruction. Take a less complex word such as *stretch*. Is my proprioceptive understanding of what you mean by the instruction *stretch* the same as yours? Likely not. We imbue our choice of words further with colour and meaning by the personal energy we bring to them and the intention with which we deliver them. They become vehicles for our energetic intention.

Starting to develop awareness of the power of words to effect physical and emotional change and to reflect on our own choices or our habitual go-to instructional words is more than half of the journey towards a holistic approach to teaching. Brainstorming your own alternatives, as I did in table 7.2, is a simple, practical exploration that will assist you in developing a teaching or self-cueing vocabulary for greater effectiveness and physical performance outcomes.

SUPPORTING AUTONOMY – CHOICES

Another key strategy for supporting the autonomy of the performer or the learner is to integrate choices into training and class planning or rehabilitation programmes. Even self-imposed training formats can involve elements of freedom and choice. The research on the impact to physical performance of introducing choices is unequivocal. This does not have to include choices as broad and consequential as those Chris Hampson offers to the Scottish Ballet dancers (see attention and focus in practice). Research suggests that even inconsequential or incidental choices promote a significant improvement in performance and effect tangible, measurable outcomes such as precision, power, jump height, speed of learning and retention. The findings relate to many kinds of skills and tasks and to all skill levels and populations. For example, when working with the senior population, increasing personal choices has been demonstrated to increase not only participants' motivation and involvement but their alertness and sense of well-being as well (Langer and Rodin 1976).

Giving inconsequential choices refers to giving choices that do not directly affect the task or learning outcome. In a study related to precision, one group of participants was allowed to choose the colour of the ball they would use, and the other group was not given a choice and the colour was imposed (Wulf, Chiviacowsky and Cardozo 2014). Logically, the colour of the ball in a precision and accuracy test is inconsequential, having no effect on the performance outcome; however, participants who were given a choice demonstrated greater speed of learning and greater accuracy. Whether you *choose* red or I *impose* red, even if you would have chosen red if given the choice, has a significant, measurable effect on performance outcome. In a similar study of incidental choice, participants about to undertake a balance test were interrupted and asked incidentally which picture they preferred to be hung on the wall in the laboratory or asked to choose the activity they would like to do after the test. Neither of these choices had any relationship with the balance test itself and yet, once again, those who had a sense of enhanced autonomy and were given choices outperformed those who did not, in terms of their fast, reflexive adjustments to balance (Lewthwaite et al. 2015).

What might we consider inconsequential or incidental choices in dance terms? There are many easy inconsequential choices that we can start to implement into dance training and rehearsal straight away, depending on

---

Attention and Focus in Practice

THE JOURNEY OF AUTONOMY

Chris Hampson, artistic director of the Scottish Ballet, choreographer, former professional dancer

Autonomy is probably the hardest element. In my mind, it's about owning the consequence, learning from it, acting with consequence, a sense of consequence and many other things. Most of the dance world functions on received wisdom and it's so rarely questioned. I think that's what I'm really wanting the dancers to do, to question the wisdom. There will be aspects that are wonderful, strong foundations, fantastic values that will never change, but we know now thankfully, publicly, there is much of that shared wisdom and shared knowledge which is really detrimental to the art form, detrimental to their own progress. That's what I'm interested in changing. So that journey of autonomy I think is really key. For example, we are doing annual appraisals at the moment; they are self-appraisals. Each dancer hands me the piece of paper and I just say 'Right, talk me through it. Let's talk about how you perceive your performance'. That's the aspiration; however, some dancers would still prefer just to know what I think!

[In terms of giving choices], the dancers now have a new health and wellness regimen. They have access to physiotherapy, chiropractic, massage, strength and conditioning, yoga, and Gyrotonics – a broad range of physical activities that support their training. So, for instance, we said to them 'That's it. Do the classes you feel you need to do'. We're not counting their classes or checking who's not jumping and who's turning. My view is, if they are doing what they need to do, they will be able to do what we require of them, and if they are not, they won't be! It gave them the permission to build their own regimen. Giving choice has worked for about two-thirds of the company. You know, we're on a journey.

the age group or skill level of the dancers. An inconsequential choice would be one that does not disturb the overall learning outcomes of your planned lesson or long-term teaching objectives, your rehearsal goals or personal goals if you are training alone. Take the example of the stickers used as an external focus in the improvised balance promenade (chapter 6). When taking this exploration with younger learners, I make sure there is always a choice of stickers – a choice between hearts or stars, for example, and lots of different colours to choose from. In fact I do this whether the dancers are beginners or professionals. Emmi (figure 6.8) chose pink hearts for the promenade. Having a choice of sticker seems to be significant, whatever the skill level! In practice, this has an immediate, noticeable effect on motivation, and research confirms the measurable effect on movement quality and outcome. Many teachers will have experienced this already when teaching young dancers who place great importance on what colour scarf they get or on being able to choose their partner dancer.

The choice may be inconsequential; however, the benefits to performance are not at all inconsequential. In a physical fitness study, one group were allowed to freely choose the order in which they completed four exercises, whilst the exercise order was imposed on the other group. Participants given this inconsequential choice demonstrated significantly increased engagement, willingness and stamina to complete more physical repetitions, approximately 40 per cent more repetitions than the participants who had the sequence order imposed on them. Now that's consequential (Wulf, Freitas and Tandy 2014).

For more advanced dancers, we might offer inconsequential choices such as Would you like to do *this* enchaînement first or the other one? To the right or to the left first? Who's starting? Do you prefer music A or B for this? Do you want to do your own stretching today or a stretch exercise with me? In rehearsal we might ask Where would you like to start? With the first excerpt or the second? Would you like to do that variation once again or is that enough for today? Inconsequential choices support the dancer's sense of autonomy and are a simple strategy for teaching staff, artistic teams and health care practitioners to implement. Consider as well to give yourself choices to boost your own training levels and maintain motivation and attention.

These research findings concur with some Eastern movement practice approaches. For example, in the practice of chi kung, we are encouraged to 'play' chi kung. Participants are actively encouraged to avoid getting attached to doing exercises in a particular fixed order, but instead to maintain a continual element of choice. This choice, as we have seen in research, encourages responsibility and motivation for our own learning and a sense of autonomy. However, the significance of play in Eastern movement practice and of incorporating choices is that it maintains a constant element of the unknown and spontaneity in practice. This element of unknown helps keep us in the present moment to revisit the ordinary with fresh eyes, in our daily practice of defamiliarization. An element of unknown heightens attentional focus and sensory listening to the present moment that enables increased energy flow and power.

More consequential choices have been demonstrated to further affect physical performance, motivation and learning (Wulf and Lewthwaite 2016). We might consider implementing some of these more consequential, evidence-based choices in our dance practice, such as allowing the dancer to have input into the extent and the pace of the practice, asking dancers whether they would like to see a skills demonstration, and asking at what point they would like to receive feedback. We could also enable dancers to identify and set their own individualized technical goals, as in the observation of videoed practice discussed in chapter 6, or we could introduce a broader personal goal-setting strategy for the dancer's self-paced learning and performance self-appraisal. These OPTIMAL elements of choice, autonomy and attentional focus promote a virtuous circle of enhanced learning and performance outcome.

ENHANCING EXPECTANCY

When we support dancers or support ourselves by boosting confidence and expectancy for high performance outcomes, we lay the groundwork for successful movement foundations. A chemical brain–body reaction occurs when we can imagine a successful outcome; dopaminergic response triggers synaptic connections to ensure the anticipated successful movement (Wulf and Lewthwaite 2016). It comes as no surprise to anyone that confidence has been established as a predictor of successful performance outcomes (Wulf and Lewthwaite 2016). Researchers Ewell and Leutgeb determine that the dopamine released contributes additionally to the consolidation of learning following successful movement attempts by boosting the replay of memories even during rest (Ewell and Leutgeb 2014). Conversely, when we lack confidence or we anticipate critique or a suboptimal or failed attempt, then dopamine is suppressed and with it the synaptic connection. Thus, movement fluidity and automaticity are undermined when confidence is lacking.

Expectancy is an adaptable concept that is illustrative of a flexible mindset. It is what a person imagines or is working towards, and the open mind means that development can be realized fluidly and faster. It is *not* the same concept as enhancing dancers' **expectations**. Expectations has a more rigid definition and means reinforcing fixed ideas that, when not fulfilled, can lead to disappointment, frustration or resentment and hinder rather than facilitate performance development (Pennell 2017). Perhaps because of this potential confusion between 'expectancy' and 'expectation' or because it feels contrary to the way in which many of us were taught, the idea of enhancing expectancy can encounter resistance in some teachers. In the pursuit of physical or artistic

---

Attention and Focus in Practice

WHEN THE ORDER IS 'CHISELED IN STONE'

Timo Kokkonen, dance educator, teacher at the Ballet School of the Finnish National Opera and Ballet, former professional dancer

I found it disturbing when learning technical steps, if someone was telling me an order which was 'chiseled in stone' and it had to be like this! Looking back, what I was taught in this traditional method just didn't work for me. When you teach small kids, you have to let them do things wrong. Teaching a saut de basque the other day the way I had been taught to teach: 'It's a battement, an à la seconde, a passé, a stretched foot', I thought, that wasn't the way I learnt it! Someone showed me, I tried to mimic it and gradually work it out myself. Ballet has been going for hundreds of years and evolved into the most economical way of working. When the body just tries things, it finds the economical way. Once you find the more or less right way, then it's easier for a teacher to fine-tune it. If something is cut into pieces too small, you can't see the whole. It's just not dance.

I remember a petit allegro section in a Nureyev Nutcracker, full of battus, 'ch ch ch ch', cou-de-pied, brisés front and back and whatever. I got it by going into a studio alone. Alone, I saw how the choreography was in the music, the music was in the choreography. They weren't just steps. I don't think it would have become so good if someone had 'taught' me and tried to give me 'the answer' of how to make it work.

I really wonder how I made it through. I was so unconscious of what I was doing. I was just 'dancing'! On the other hand, it worked! Maybe it's better not to be so conscious about it – because then it was dance.

---

excellence there is a natural tendency to focus only on what's not right, to highlight the faults and to offer feedback frequently following failed attempts. With this well-meaning fault-finding approach, however, we further undermine confidence and suppress dopamine production, which leads to less-than-optimal movement and further failed attempts that consolidate expectancy of failure in a self-perpetuating downward spiral. The performance expectancy of a dancer can be supported proactively in several ways or, alternatively, can be supported by mitigating perceived difficulty and effort to build solid confidence and performance foundations.

A priority focus on identifying the positive elements of a performance, the 'keepers' (perhaps identified by the dancers themselves), creates the building blocks for a resilient performing foundation. We might also systematically target task-specific feedback following only the *positive* attempts rather than giving feedback after the failed attempts as might be more habitual. Research shows that feedback given following successful attempts has a greater impact on both performance outcome and retention of learning (Chiviacowsky and Wulf 2007; Chiviacowsky et al. 2009). (See chapter 8 for optimal attentional cueing.)

When performance psychologists refer to enhancing expectancy, they are often referring to what is termed *social comparative feedback* – for example, that participants are performing better than average for their age or for their age group or compared to other similar classes or groups. This kind of social comparative feedback is shown to enhance movement efficiency and speed of mastery and promote a greater stamina and tolerance for effort (Wulf and Lewthwaite 2016). Social comparative feedback is particularly effective with younger children (Saemi et al. 2011). In a dance context, this might be motivational feedback such as 'Well done! You've got that really well. I don't think even the grade 8s could do that!' *Thinking* that we are doing well or are being effective or efficient means that we *become* more effective or efficient (Stoate and Wulf 2011). In my own practice experience, this approach of enhancing expectancy also works well to facilitate movement fluency in older adult dancers and those with special needs; however, exaggerated social-comparative feedback is not recommended for the preprofessional or professional dancer. We can't imagine saying 'You've grasped that section so much quicker than any other Lilac Fairy!' Enhancing expectancies with exaggeration would be questionable at a professional level and could erode the relationship of trust and confidence an artist must develop with their coach. The need to support the confidence and autonomy of the artist, however, remains at all skills levels and can be approached using other strategies to enhance expectancy.

ENHANCING EXPECTANCY – MITIGATING PERCEIVED DIFFICULTY

Another approach to enhancing expectancy is to become aware of how we as teachers or coaches transmit, often inadvertently, our own perceived difficulty of the task. This can happen in many subtle ways, from the wording of instructions and the tone of voice adopted to other nonverbal indicators of effort. Instructions might preempt and transmit perceived difficulty or effort like this: 'Now, you'll find this more challenging; it's a difficult phrase.' Or indicate difficulty through the tone of the voice, 'Ha, ha. Now let's try that on the *other* side', where the derisive laugh and tone of voice could indicate that the other side will be more challenging and introduce the idea of possible failure. Teachers can also transmit inappropriate effort and communicate difficulty through nonverbal means such as drawing breath in through the teeth in preparation, 'And adage . . . tsphffffff . . . and one'. Nonverbal transmission of the perceived difficulty of an exercise or movement can be as subtle as the teacher holding their breath as they prepare, raising the eyebrows or folding the arms in a particular way. These small gestures transmit accurately a teacher's own mindset and pass on to dancers a multidimensional 'hologram' of appropriate effort and energy or even of fear and holding as they embark on the exercise. As a dancer, we can perpetuate this received or perceived difficulty in our own self-talk, inadvertently undermining further the potential success of our movements.

Simply determining to underplay the difficulty of the task or mitigate the learner's perceived difficulty is a constructive strategy for enhancing dancers' expectancies. Older adults, for example, who would typically display impaired reactivity and stability in balance tests, showed significantly improved stability and long-term recall of acquired balance skills when given the feedback 'active people like you can normally get this exercise quite easily' (Wulf, Chiviacowsky and Lewthwaite 2012). In dance, this positive underplaying of the difficulty might sound something like 'Let's work on the allegro section. You'll grasp the dynamics easily'.

ENHANCING EXPECTANCY – REDEFINING SUCCESS

A sense of success is a necessary component for speeding the consolidation of learning and to achieving mastery of movement (Trempe, Sabourin and Proteau 2012). Research shows that when the definition of success or the definition of a narrowly defined goal is relaxed a little, the participants' accuracy and speed of learning are greatly enhanced. In figure 7.1, the golf hole is an analogy for a narrow definition of success. Rather than success being defined as 'the golf hole and nothing else', the definition could be opened up a little and described as 'anywhere in the bigger circle will be great'. As a direct impact of this broader definition of success, participants' speed of learning and accuracy to achieve the narrower desired goal, the golf hole, is increased. When success is narrowly defined, many unsuccessful attempts will be experienced that reinforce a sense of failure, further undermining future performance outcome.

The technical demands of dance are such that both dancers and teachers tend to focus only on the narrow definition of success, the desired perfect end goal: the perfect pirouette position or the perfect arabesque line or the perfect jump form. The definition of the movement objectives in dance are

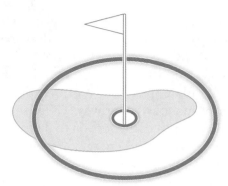

Figure 7.1   Using a golf hole as an analogy for a narrow definition of success or failure. A sense of initial success is experienced with a broader goal or more relaxed movement objective (outer circle) that accelerates speed of learning to mastery of the narrower, desired, real goal or movement objective (inner circle).

precise and unforgiving, like the golf hole. Ensuing teacher feedback might be predominantly focused on the faults of the many unsuccessful attempts, 'No, not like that', reinforcing the fact that all attempts falling short of the perfect goal are experienced as failures by the learner.

Consider that by broadening the definition of success – the definition of the goal or movement objective – learners can experience a small sense of initial success, which consolidates confidence, triggers dopamine and speeds their ability to master the perfect desired movement objective. For example, in a sustained phrase that requires strength and adaptability for balance, we might suggest 'This balance sustains right through the six-count phrase; however, if you can sustain through four counts for now and then tombé, that will be great'.

These findings may feel counterintuitive to some teachers. However, if we clearly describe the desired perfect objective and then open up our definition of success, then our teaching will be more effective, allowing learners to experience an initial sense of success that lays the foundation for them to effectively achieve our real movement objective.

CUMULATIVE EFFECT

Although these new considerations and strategies might seem like a lot to take on board at first, the good news is that they can be introduced one at a time as and when you have chance to experiment with them in class. The benefits of introducing such strategies are cumulative. As you incorporate them into your practice, the benefits to performance outcome and learning increase incrementally (Chua, Wulf and Lewthwaite 2018). That is to say that the more you are able to integrate them into your teaching practice, the more effective your teaching will be. So whether you choose first to

- develop and integrate the use of external attentional focus,
- become aware of your teaching language and choice of vocabulary,
- determine to enhance dancers' performance expectancies and mitigate the difficulty and effort involved or
- implement choice systematically into class planning,

these complementary approaches support one another in a virtuous circle that increases the dancers' sense of self-efficacy and ensures that the *desired* movement objectives and *actual* movement execution are aligned.

Perhaps begin with just one element that attracts your interest and seems 'doable' and explore ways to integrate that into class delivery and planning, and then move on to another in any order you want. It's like learning a new language and takes a conscious choice to implement, particularly because it's not the way that most of us were trained. Be kind to yourself as you experiment – practical application of the new 'language' will lead to fluency.

From a dancer's perspective, we can do a lot by bringing our attention to the potentially controlling language that we use in self-talk and self-cueing and to the perceived difficulty we perpetuate that can make us preempt and anticipate difficulty. We can develop awareness of the perceptions of effort we hold or have learnt that might predetermine a less-than-optimal outcome. As dancers, we are renowned for our discipline and determination. However, allowing some freedom of choice or spontaneity in self-training programmes or in the planning of daily routines can promote unexpected enhanced physical benefits such as strength, stamina and speed of learning.

From a professional, multidisciplinary team perspective at The Royal Ballet, we've explored a united approach to autonomy support and external attentional focus in a rehearsal scenario. With a principal dancer, artistic rehearsal director and health care team working together, we aimed to

- be attentive to the wording of instructions, using open and supportive wording,
- offer hints and suggestions rather than demands and commands,
- support autonomy through choices and
- promote a consistent, external attentional focus throughout.

These holistic approaches function cumulatively to promote a cohesive, dancer-centric language from all team members.

The result is not only that the dancer experiences improved technical facility and greater physical ease, but also the united language and intention of the team supports the dancer to sustain their optimal attentional focus, free of conscious movement-control thinking. Freeing up cognitive reserve, the dancer experiences a greater capacity to recall multidisciplinary information as needed and an improved sensory perception to hear and respond to the live pianist *and* to retain additional on-the-spot artistic and therapeutic feedback *whilst* dancing. A united team approach facilitates the interdisciplinary team skills of collaboration, communication and listening that support the dancer in the global demands of the discipline whilst still allowing the space and the freedom for individual interpretation and artistry.

Choreographer William Forsythe, for example, also consciously supports the autonomy of the dancers by giving them choices and having the intention that dancers connect their own joy and motivation for dance to the work. He shares this in a video from The National Ballet of Canada on physical thinking.

> I want the dancers to say something. I'd like them to connect with *why* they are dancing, which usually has to do with something they love. They have tremendous desire and love of dancing otherwise they couldn't survive in an environment that demands so much, so I try to give them something that respects that desire. (National Ballet of Canada 2019)

REFLECTION PROMPTS

The field of performance psychology that promotes state-of-the-art strategies for mindful training to enhance performance outcome and motivation for learning is a vast field of study. This chapter merely touches on some elements that contribute to the success of learning and performance to put attention and focus into a broader context. As we dancers, teachers, choreographers and artistic directors bring our attention to *how* we deliver information and not simply attend to the *what* – the *content* of that information to be delivered – then technique and artistry will be liberated and performance heightened incrementally.

- If you decide to start with awareness of the teaching **language**, perhaps begin by observing other instructors teaching and identify some of their choices. Is their tone predominantly controlling or supportive of the dancers? Jot down a few phrases that you hear. What are the words that come up repeatedly? If they are controlling instructions, how would you word those instructions differently? Are there small modifications you could make that would allow the dancers more of a sense of autonomy, a sense of freedom? Could you adapt some of the commands to make them into suggestions or tips for the dancers, for example? Write a few alternative phrasings for yourself based on the original phrases to inspire your own teaching practice or self-cueing language.

- Did you notice anything happen in your body in exploration 7.1 when you changed between the two instruction words? Were there changes to the muscular tension you used? The amount of effort? A change in the breathing perhaps? Or a change in the focus? A sense of space, of freedom, of dancing? A change in the wording can bring new lightness, energy or focus to a movement. Perhaps create a list like table 7.2 and collect the vocabulary that you frequently use when you cue yourself or when you teach others. Be as creative and inventive as you like and brainstorm alternative instructional vocabulary that you might use. If you are unsure about a word, try a quick comparison exploration in movement as we did to feel the potential qualities or the sense of flow and space that the new word allows.

- If you teach, you can develop your awareness of these motivational strategies by recording one of your classes (audio recording is enough). Listen to it quietly later and focus on some of the choices you made, consciously or unconsciously, in class. Try to detach yourself as you listen, as if simply observing another teacher working.

  - How is the overall tone of the language used? To what extent are you using commands – could you word some of those differently to support autonomy?

  - Does the class offer possibilities for choice to the learner? What kind of inconsequential choices are you already incorporating into class?

  - Can you hear whether you inadvertently transmit a sense of difficulty as you describe the tasks? When do you seem to do that? With power and stamina tasks (allegro)? Dynamic balance tasks (pirouette)? In speed? Or sustained balance (adage)? Is it your own perceived difficulty about the task that you are transmitting?

Just becoming aware of *how* we share information, of potential transfer that preempts difficulty, will be the first step on the journey to doing things differently and to finding creative alternatives to support learning and the developing artist.

CHAPTER 8

OPTIMAL ATTENTIONAL CUEING

You have to be open to correction, be open to not knowing . . . you have to channel the desire to expand yourself in order to make it, and then again even when you are professional, in order to be an artist.

Susan Jaffe, former principal dancer, American Ballet Theater (Thomson 2018)

Now that you've created a space for attention to your everyday practice – to the familiar movement patterns, your habitual choices, the received wisdom, your stream of interfering thoughts, your intentions and unconscious transmission, and to the ceaseless nature of universal energy – you've allowed a space in your dance for quantum change to occur. That creative space between the conscious thoughts – that no-mind state – is a product of bringing your attention and focus to the quality, effect or pathway of your movement and to your sensations in the moment. The philosopher Osho describes this state of moving with complete attention in the moment: The whole awareness and energy shifts to the movement, which becomes 'full', and conversely the mind becomes free of thought and spacious. There's no energy left for thinking, he declares (Osho n.d.).

This mirrors the fascinating exchanges I've had with Dr Hanna Poikonen to summarize, from a neuroscientific perspective, that when we are thinking, consciously interfering or attempting to control or adjust our own body parts or body movement, our performance cannot be optimal. It will not be fluid nor efficient, it will be uneconomic and inconsistent, and we'll experience diminished capacity for sensory perception and multitasking. If we are in *this* place, we are predominantly functioning in the primary motor cortex, which hinders fluid, masterful movement (Poikonen 2020). As a teacher or coach, our choice of attentional focus then might retain the dancer, forcing them to constantly 'think' about their own body and consistently bring them back to the primary motor cortex. Becoming aware of this attentional process and drawing the dancers' attention far from conscious thought enables access to other neural networks that are essential for more fluid, economic and autonomous movement (Poikonen 2020).

As a teacher or therapist, opportunities to draw dancers away from the temptation to think about body-part control can be achieved through the deliberate focus and structuring of our instruction, feedback and cueing. As a dancer, we can guide our own attention by using an optimal self-cueing format. Until we consciously develop our own repertoire of effective cues that resonate personally, self-cues and teaching feedback will tend to be formulated in the language we hear or we heard from our teachers and coaches. So let's take a practical look at how we can structure information in a dance context to harness our attention and allow for that space in our dance that enables our power, precision and artistry to flourish.

The objective of feedback is to provide information about a person's performance of a task that can be used as the basis for further improvement and learning. A cue is simply a prompt or reminder that focuses the attention (Lexicon n.d.). Feedback coming from an outside source, a teacher or a recording is referred to as *extrinsic* or *augmented feedback* and is balanced by the sensory information, or intrinsic feedback, that dancers gather by sensing, feeling, hearing or seeing their own performance (LeBorgne and Daniels Rosenberg 2021).

STRUCTURING OPTIMAL FEEDBACK

Today in dance classes, many teachers try to give positive, supportive feedback to dancers in order, I believe, to proactively change the traditional dance learning environment predominantly made up of fault finding and negative feedback or the alternative stony silence that many of us grew up in. This initiative includes, in large part, motivational words or statements such as 'Great!', 'Bravo!', 'Well done', 'Gorgeous!', 'Much better'. This is a fantastic initiative for improving the ambience of class or rehearsal; however, strictly speaking this is not feedback. It's an evaluation or value judgement that contains little or no actionable information. Dancers might feel momentarily happy, if the praise is sincere, that someone appreciated what they did, but they will have not learnt anything (Wiggins 2012; Rist 2001).

So how can we build on these motivational statements and structure them optimally to focus attention and support effective learning? One simple suggestion is to imagine punctuation after the motivational statement, such as a comma or colon, that reminds us to continue with task-specific information relating to the performance – for example, 'Much better: . . .' Another suggestion is using the dancer's name. This simple, obvious addition will enhance the reception of the task-specific information that follows (Wiggins 2012; Rist 2001).

When structuring task-specific information, aim to promote an external focus of attention at all times and draw the dancer's focus to the quality, effect, trajectory or sensory aspects of the movement to take advantage of all the performance and learning benefits we have explored so far. For optimal reception and reaction by brain–body pathways, these external focus feedback statements need to be **positively formulated**.

POSITIVELY VERSUS NEGATIVELY FORMULATED

In my experience, there is a misunderstanding among many teachers regarding the definition of *positively formulated*. It does not mean that we should simply compliment the dancer all the time – That was super, darling! – and ignore what needs improvement. *Positive* in this context means that the statement should contain concrete information or personalized observation about the performance or advice about the desired action. The opposite, *negatively formulated* feedback, highlights only the *undesirable* action observed (Wegner et al. 1987; Rathle 2018). For example, 'Don't drop the foot' is negatively formulated IF feedback that highlights what is *not* desirable and offers no alternative, actionable information. Alternative feedback advice for the same performance result might be 'That was very low. Push down against the ground and spiral open',

'Make a clear triangle' or 'Feel the touch of your shoe'. These are positively formulated EF feedback statements that provide actionable information and advice about the movement we *would* like to achieve (Rathle 2018).

The analogy I like to use for the process of learning movement skills is that of creating a personal road map to guide your movement. Imagine that rather than dancing, you are driving a car and waiting for feedback. You're driving along quite fast, which is a little scary because you've no idea where you are going. When I say 'Whatever you do, don't turn right!' you think 'OK, but I still have no idea which direction I'm supposed to go'. There is no information for your mental road map. As we learn, we piece together concrete information about our performance, both from extrinsic and intrinsic feedback. We reaffirm and store positively formulated information or key milestones that become building blocks in our acquisition of that skill. Negatively formulated statements are simply a 'void' of information that give no concrete input for the dancer who is left 'driving' in the dark.

Although negatively formulated feedback is frequently employed in dance teaching – Remember don't do. . . . No! Not like that. – it actually cannot be computed by our neural structure (Wegner et al. 1987). Our attention is always drawn to the concrete or positive part of the information, in this case, to the very action that is *not* desirable in the movement. When we hear 'Don't bend your knees', the information that our brain can register is 'Bend your knees'. You must have heard the metaphorical illustration 'Don't think of a pink elephant', and as soon as you hear this instruction, all you can think of *is* a pink elephant because you have no other concrete information that would focus your attention elsewhere. According to research, in the absence of alternative positively formulated information, these negatively formulated statements reinforce precisely the movement patterns that we want to progress. So, the instruction 'Don't lift your shoulders' (IF) or 'Don't lift like that' (EF), whether they have an internal or external focus, will result in *more* lifting of the shoulders rather than in any improvement of the movement form. This makes negatively formulated feedback doubly counterproductive for teaching (Rathle 2018; Wegner et al. 1987). The format for effective feedback advice focuses on what *can* be achieved and delivers simple blocks of affirmative information that the dancer can piece together into a clear road map that is embedded in new neural pathways.

OPTIMAL FORMAT

When developing effective feedback, it is recommended to stick to the FACTS. Ensure that it's formative, actionable, clear, timely and supportive (Brigham Young University n.d.; Wiggins 2012).

Formative: The feedback focuses on the observed task at hand and the identified learning objectives or learning outcomes for that task rather than randomly addressing many aspects of overall performance at once. It is personalized and specific to a performer or group.

Actionable: The feedback should be concrete and tangible. I love the example of ballet master Sorella Englund of The Royal Danish Ballet, who recalls the kind of artistic feedback she was given early in her performing career, 'Try to be your unconsciousness together with your consciousness!' This is neither tangible nor actionable. As an artist, she realized the importance of a clear one-thing-at-a-time approach to feedback, which she says she is still developing to this day with the help of the dancers and artists who are now *her* teachers (Englund 2019).

Clear: The feedback information should be understandable, easy to implement, transparent, and above all, it should be dancer centric and aimed at supporting the performer, rather than formulated in an idiosyncratic way that only the teacher, therapist or choreographer can understand. Without conscious attention to the language of feedback, when teaching a large class with lots of material to get through we frequently reach for easy-access words and descriptors that are unclear. Ambiguous descriptors that we hear a lot in dance: 'That was a *beautiful* line', 'a *nice* developpé', 'Give me *pretty* footwork', 'Reach the *correct* position', 'Make a *proper* finish'. These easy descriptors are subjective and open to interpretation. This means that the feedback is unclear to the learner and therefore ineffective. Alternative words you could use to complete those feedback statements that would carry clear, concrete information include fluid, extending, high, smooth, never-ending, sharp, percussive, grounded, crossed, open, closed, fast, tight, abrupt or melting. The brainstorming of potential vocabulary from exploration 7.1 is a great support and provides alternative, effective words for in-the-moment choices in class.

Remember that feedback is not limited to verbal delivery. Nonverbal feedback such as sounds, facial expressions and gestures that teachers and coaches use may also be unclear, leaving dancers in the dark about what they need to do to improve. Education specialist Dr Grant Wiggins suggests recording classes regularly and observing or listening to our own in-the-moment choices. He suggests that self-observation is a transformative experience for a teacher or coach. Concepts and verbal and nonverbal feedback, or gestures that appeared crystal clear at the time, can seem obscure and confusing when we observe them later and, importantly, we can see the reaction of dancers and students that we might not have picked up on at the time (Wiggins 2012).

Timely and Supportive: One of the most important aspects of effective feedback is the timing and consistency of delivery – when is feedback information best placed for optimum reception and integration by the learner? How much feedback should we be giving to enhance results? Systematic feedback frequency and optimal timing are further enhanced by the tone of the language we choose as we explored in chapter 7, by our underlying intention and the extent to which our language supports a sense of autonomy in learning. We'll look at the timing

TABLE 8.1   Examples of Optimal Feedback Structure

MOTIVATION OR EVALUATION	POSITIVELY FORMULATED PERFORMANCE FEEDBACK	PRESCRIPTION OR ADVICE
Bravo, Greg:	Really strong attack	*Next time see if you can shift the orientation to take in the audience.*
Beautiful, Sylvie:	Smooth, sustained unfolding. The line is still low.	*Now press down and focus on the direction of the diagonal line.*
Yes, better Fran:	Good strong push downwards.	*Next time see if you can push into all five directions.*

and frequency of effective feedback in the next sections on feedback delivery: Delivering Optimal Feedback and Optimal Feedback Quantity for Performance Enhancement.

What we typically refer to as feedback actually comprises several elements: (1) motivation, evaluation or value judgement; (2) concrete, formative information about the observed performance; and (3) prescriptive feedback or advice aimed at the progression of technique or the desired artistic objectives. For this three-part feedback to be effective, be selective and concise with your choice of words, images and gestures and take a one-thing-at-a-time approach to provide clear milestones for the dancers' mental road map. It's essential, from a neuroscientific perspective, to support the dancers' attention and focus and not overload them with diverse information that will disable neural networks and cause further deterioration to performance and learning.

Table 8.1 offers examples of a concise structure for optimal feedback that the brain can easily register and that promotes effective neuromuscular functioning and reaction. In shorthand, the structure might be described as follows:

motivation or evaluation and name: + what I observed (**+** *advice*)

This clear two- or three-part structuring of feedback elements facilitates optimal reception, attention, reaction and, therefore, progression of learning.

Although our first reaction as a teacher might be 'I've no time whilst teaching to implement such a feedback structure', consider that 'no time for feedback' actually translates to 'no time to promote learning' (Wiggins 2012). Once you know your students or the performers, then this concise feedback structure need not take so much time. You can use minimal well-chosen words, and you can achieve a lot with clear, nonverbal feedback whilst the rest of the class or rehearsal continues. Let's take a look at the feedback:

Yes, better Fran: Good strong push downwards. *Next time, see if you can push into all five directions.*

If you are under a lot of time pressure and with an experienced dancer that you know well, this might even take the form of 100 per cent nonverbal feedback:

Eye contact with Fran. Enthusiastic nodding and big smile. Clear, vertical pushing down gesture plus an affirmative thumbs up. Uplifting, extending gesture radiating in all directions like a star. Eye contact again plus a short concluding smile or nod of the head to indicate end of feedback. This took no more than 10 seconds.

Choose whatever form or mixture of verbal and nonverbal feedback works best in your dance context and is the most clear and easy to apply for the specific age group, skill level and ability of the dancers.

DELIVERING OPTIMAL FEEDBACK

In dance, teachers rarely consciously consider the most appropriate or optimal timing to deliver their feedback observations as part of a strategy for maximum feedback effect. In a traditionally teacher-centric and fault-finding discipline, it is tempting to jump in with feedback immediately as soon as we spot some undesirable aspect of performance. However, extensive research shows that this is not the most effective moment to deliver feedback to learners. The best feedback is **timely**, not immediate (Wiggins 2012). When observing a task or an action multiple times, the most effective strategy is to remain quiet and observe further, resisting the impulse to jump in with immediate feedback advice. The most effective strategy is to place the feedback information deliberately after the *best* of several repetitions rather than after the first or the worst (Chiviacowsky and Wulf 2007). Children as young as six years old, when shown videos (extrinsic feedback) of their own *best* trial out of several, demonstrate more ability to improve their movement form and quality than children who are shown their *average* performance (Clark and Ste-Marie 2007).

Although, as a teacher, you might find yourself *biting your tongue*, this later placement following a slightly better result promotes superior reception of feedback information and advice. It therefore improves brain–body reaction and integration of feedback and retention, enhancing progression at all skill levels and with all age groups (Chiviacowsky and Wulf 2007; Chiviacowsky et al. 2009; Saemi et al. 2011).

In another study, performers were asked to choose when they would like to receive their feedback. The performers determined when they would find it most supportive and helpful to receive information and advice as opposed to having it imposed on them according to the timing of the teacher or rehearsal director. Participants given the choice requested feedback after better trials and showed enhanced ability to improve the movement based on that feedback information. Participants who had no choice about when they received their feedback did not make as much progress in comparison, and when asked, they reported that they would have preferred feedback after their more positive attempts (Chiviacowsky and Wulf 2002). The enhanced sense of autonomy provided when a performer is given the *choice* of when to receive feedback information, as we explored in chapter 7, is shown to further improve performance results.

Perhaps due to time constraints or to the sheer quantity of teaching content, many teachers find themselves delivering verbal feedback right at the end of an exercise or even at the end of the class with a quick 'Next time, remember . . .' before moving swiftly on. Feedback given without providing the opportunity to put it into practice and allow performers to embody and register it on their road map is a wasted learning opportunity and is wasted breath for the teacher. Particularly in movement learning, concepts that remain at a cognitive level in the brain are challenging to retain and are quickly lost. Certain choreographers similarly give reams of notes and 'download' large amounts of feedback right at the end of a rehearsal or performance. Give performers the opportunity to implement the new information and actively reshape their performance (Wiggins 2012; Brigham Young University n.d.; Rathle 2018; Glasstone 1991). Hold back and save the feedback observation and advice for the next practical class or rehearsal.

As we have seen already when promoting an external attentional focus or developing autonomy supportive language or observing our own nonverbal transmission, it's our intention and *how* we say or do something that is the most significant factor. So using a supportive tone is the 'S' of the feedback FACTS (Brigham Young University n.d.; Wiggins 2012). When feedback is delivered in a supportive and understanding way, learners are more open to receive it and more able to build on that external guidance. Intention and tone then are the make-or-break aspects of effective teaching for the reception of well-structured feedback advice (Brigham Young University n.d.).

Optimal feedback can be summarized as follows:

- It is ongoing and ideally consistently placed after better repetitions or when the performer chooses to receive it.

- It uses supportive language that is formatted using a positively formulated, two- or three-part structure of EF information (**motivation** + observation + *advice*) that facilitates dancers' attention and focus to enhance the movement outcome.

- It allows dancers time to implement new information immediately so they can effectively process, embody and register key learning milestones on their personal movement road map.

OPTIMAL FEEDBACK QUANTITY FOR PERFORMANCE ENHANCEMENT

There is a general assumption that too much feedback is not helpful to learners and could make them dependent on an external eye (Wulf et al. 2010). This generalization assumes that the elements involved in external feedback – motivation and evaluation, performance observation and prescriptive advice – all have the same potential effect on performance and performers. Let's take a look at these elements one by one.

Motivational or evaluational feedback (1) is an important element in a positive learning environment and can encourage a mindset for growth and development. However, if it is used excessively it can lose its sincerity and, therefore, its impact. A potential 'dark side' of excessive external motivation is a learner's gradual dependence on the praise. The dancer works to receive teachers' compliments and approval rather than focusing on the process of personal growth or the personal desire to improve that is essential for building the necessary resilience in such a demanding discipline (Meadows-Fernandez 2017; Karin and Nordin-Bates 2019).

The **concrete, formative information** (2) that we share following an observed performance is shown to impact learning and results more in function of the attentional focus that the feedback information promotes, rather than through any particular optimum prescribed frequency for that performance information (Wulf et al. 2010). As we have explored in earlier chapters, if feedback guides attention towards the self and encourages the dancer to consciously adjust a body part and interfere with their performance, then *more* of this internal focus-inducing feedback degrades movement efficiency and accuracy further, the more it is applied. Conversely, findings show that performance feedback that is structured to promote an external focus further enhances performance the *more* it is delivered. In a study, EF feedback given 100 per cent of the time, that is to say after every repetition, promoted greater benefits to performance results than in trials when EF feedback was given less frequently, only after every third repetition. So, in terms of performance feedback, when we guide and sustain the dancers' attention on the movement quality, trajectory or objective, then more feedback produces better results (Wulf et al. 2010).

Lastly, giving a high ratio of **prescriptive feedback advice** (3) relative to observed performance information (2) *is* thought to be detrimental to learning. Continually providing external advice and external solutions to movement challenges, however well meaning, can discourage learners from developing trust in their own intrinsic feedback and from engaging their own judgement, which is essential for personal development and progression of learning. The need for a developed foundation of trust in one's own intrinsic feedback process and in one's own judgement is important when a dancer receives conflicting advice from different external sources or from different disciplines, for example, which is a common occurrence. Dancers moving from a preprofessional to a professional company environment also frequently find themselves plunged into the situation where external advice is suddenly no longer available to them at all. So balancing the ratio of teacher-fed prescriptive advice (3) with the implementation of other strategies for interactive learning and solution finding is essential for the development of this intrinsic process (Wiggins 2012; Wulf et al. 2010).

Are you aware of your own ratio of feedback advice and solutions (3) to performance observation feedback (2) that you offer in teaching? Take the opportunity to review the teaching recordings you made in chapters 6 and 7 and look for your habitual feedback patterns. If you give a lot of prescriptive advice (3), see if you could do that differently and find ways to engage the dancers directly in their own solution finding. This could be as simple as asking them, 'Given the feedback observation (2), what do you suggest you might do or change?' (Wiggins 2012). As in the example of videoing students' work for goal setting (chapter 6), performers can usually self-advise or self-prescribe quite incisively if given the opportunity and the practice. Developing such possibilities for integrative learning, questioning and self-sought solutions in class or in rehearsal supports the autonomy of the performers and increases their motivation and ownership of the learning process and promotes an exponential increase in learning (Lambert 2012).

If the idea of implementing such a systematic approach to feedback seems daunting at first during precious class time, start simply by bringing your attention to your current feedback choices. You might add the dancer's name if you don't do that already and imagine the mental punctuation after the motivational feedback to establish the idea of a progression of feedback information. With the conscious decision to expand your skills and your practice and the encouraging experience of dancers' improved speed of learning, it will soon become a reflex to complete the feedback information. Allowing that space in your dance practice to observe your own processes and to be 'open to not knowing', as Susan Jaffe recommends (Thomson 2018, para. 10), opens the pathway for exponential change.

CUEING ATTENTION FOR HIGH PERFORMANCE

Cueing for high performance, whether self-cueing or coaching, is an art rarely taught as part of dance training. It is *not*, as so frequently seen, simply an extension of the class and rehearsal feedback process. Many choreographers and teachers give feedback information right up until the curtain goes up

Attention and Focus in Practice

KNOW YOUR BODY'S POSSIBILITIES AND LIMITATIONS

Madeleine Onne, artistic director of the Finnish National Ballet, coach, teacher, former professional dancer

Because of my back, a rather severe scoliosis, I knew I had limitations. The only thing I thought was to keep as straight as possible and focus on getting everything in and up. When turning, I was 'straight' because I could always find something in the room straight to focus on.

Energy inspired me. Some teachers came into the room and it was like an injection; their energy just took over. I try to give that energy when I'm teaching allegro, for example, because when people think it's fun, they're jumping faster and higher without really knowing it!

I never really analyzed steps. I'm always saying 'Don't think so much.' 'Close your eyes.' 'What is your body *feeling*?' 'Where is your weight?' Dancers seem to have stopped 'feeling' where they *are*, where their centre is. They want answers to everything. How should I do this? Why doesn't it work? Why, why, why? As a teacher, I try to answer as much as I can, but after all these questions, dancers try to piece it all together and find they can't move! That's why I suggest to *feel* your body. Our bodies are so different. If I tell A what she should do, that doesn't work for B. Look at me with my crooked back. I could *not* do the things or put my weight the same way as someone else. I couldn't lift my legs according to the book. I had to figure it out. How does it work with *my* body? You need to find out what works for you. Of course, dancers need guidance and the outside eye sees a lot! The trick is to *combine* that information with your own feeling and knowledge of your body's possibilities and limitations.

(Rathle 2018) (see Englund's attention and focus in practice later in this chapter). Although this may be well intentioned, it's a director- or teacher-centric action, and it is not supportive of the high-performance needs of the dancer. Overloading information, particularly at this moment, will simply block neural networks and seriously undermine performance results. It's not neurologically possible to carry a whole performance, competition or examination to cue yourself to be wonderful to

- be in an optimum physical and mental condition,
- be 100 per cent present, alert and ready with heightened senses to react to any in-the-moment eventuality and

- 'speak' through the body to communicate your artistry,

whilst simultaneously trying to recall the 25 last-minute things that are still 'not good enough' (Englund 2019). No one can perform at their optimum when fragmented in this way.

The art of high-performance cueing, whether we look at it from a sport science perspective, a neuroscientific perspective or from the perspective of the ancient teachings of Eastern movement practice, is the art of supporting a no-mind state in movement. This desired state, in which the mind is quiet and free from distracting self-related thought and judgement and 100 per cent present, is an essential factor of optimum physical and mental performance that permits maximum cognitive reserve for in-the-moment reaction and artistic interpretation.

Performance cues in high-level sports, for example, are defined as personal, positive and short (Hedstrom 2014). They are clear, brief statements, images or proprioceptive sensations, worded to prompt an external focus of attention and enhance performance results. They guide the mind, helping to keep self-related thoughts at bay and prevent the 'choking', or freezing, effect that is known to occur when thinking about one's own actions (Benz et al. 2016; Wulf 2007).

It's important that the chosen external focus cue word, statement or image has personal relevance and is an element within the performer's control for it to become an effective performance tool – an anchor for the mind. It should inspire and motivate and also encapsulate and consolidate essential information about the desired form, quality, dynamics or movement effect. Examples from sports tend to be pared down to the absolute minimum, so for instance, in a study of long-distance runners, single-word cues were used for each of the different stages of the race such as 'push' and reach (the 'heel') and 'claw' to guide their attention (Poirier Leroy n.d.). In a survey of martial arts performers, on the other hand, they tended to use a single descriptive word for each movement or movement phrase such as 'drive, cut, fast, explode' as Hanshaw and Sukal found (quoted in Hanshaw 2018), more as we might imagine doing in dance.

The attentional focus study of professional classical dancers revealed a general absence of an attentional focus and cueing strategy in the majority of participants (Guss-West and Wulf 2016). Much of the chosen self-cueing was long and loaded with feedback information and advice, evoking multiple, potentially conflicting foci. Dancers described cueing themselves for challenging movements with a list of body-related corrections such as 'square shoulders and hips, pulling up on the supporting leg', 'hold the back straight and lift the arabesque as high as possible', 'lifting my belly button to engage my abdominals'. Some even used negatively formulated cues such as the well intentioned 'look forward to the turning; *don't* worry about it' or the disabling 'focus on *not* turning in my back foot in fourth position' (Guss-West and Wulf 2016). With such self-focused attentional cueing, we undermine our own best efforts and cannot discover our highest capabilities or our own personal best.

A few dancers in the study did demonstrate examples of conscious, positively formulated supportive cueing, whether intuitively or studied, to enhance their performance. These dancers used personalized cues such as 'Powering into it – finding stillness and breadth – turnout and suspend', 'Push the limits of an imaginary circle', 'Lifting up from centre . . . feeling the length in the movement', 'Juicy plié in preparation'. There were positive motivational cues such as 'Keeping it as simple and relaxed as possible' and 'Push into the floor – let the rest happen by itself' and inspirational, minimalist cues such as 'Trajectory height and space' and 'Reach for the sky' (Guss-West and Wulf 2016).

The longer the duration of performance, the more important a cueing strategy is because the mind has time to wander as a result of fatigue and stress or time for distractions from other elements of the performance or other performers (Poirier Leroy n.d.). In longer, more challenging sequences, multiple, brief, external focus cues can be used for each movement as in the martial arts example. These can be grouped or themed serially so that as a performer you can create your own performing logic, a kind of cueing 'film' or story board (Wulf 2013). During less challenging choreographic moments, you might use a single, simple cue word or image per phrase of movement, such as 'music', 'partner', 'energy' or 'enjoy', or you may find that a single cue suffices to sustain the focus of attention through a whole variation or choreographic section. (See Englund 2019, attention and focus in practice.)

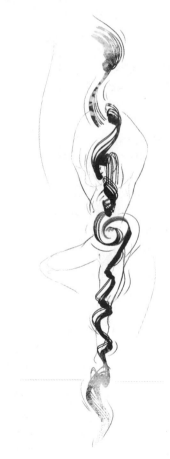

Figure 8.1   Using energy flow as a clear, concise self-cue. 'Imagining the energy flowing – It's clearer and simpler for my mind to process' (Kaba 2019).

PEAK PERFORMANCE STATE

In dance, some coaches and teachers are intuitively aware of the impact of what they might say (or refrain from saying) just before a performance can have on the performance outcome for the dancer. At that point of performance, we have to trust that the feedback is 'in there' and allow space for performance alchemy and artistry. It's the mark of high-performers to be able to select and practice their own preferred approach to promote this no-mind state prior to performance to guide the mind. Dancer Drew Hedditch describes the sensory focus of his performance preparation in The Australian Ballet's video *Ballet Anatomy: Eyes*.

> I tend to close my eyes before I go on and listen to the orchestra. Every-thing is so dark . . . when you're out there . . . all the intricate muscles coming into play whilst your eyes regather. (Australian Ballet 2018)

Performers of many disciplines describe this same phenomenon as a Zen-like state in which you drop out of the conscious level of thinking to a lower level where everything happens much faster (Wulf 2007). This no-mind state is a dynamic balance and requires consistent attention throughout performance, not just preperformance, particularly before challenging movement sequences or variations. Physical movement together with the presence of a public and their constant evaluation of our performance are factors that are known to make us particularly susceptible to self-consciousness and self-related thought. When our attention suddenly shifts to our self and consciousness of our own performance, we open the pathway for other debilitating, random thoughts and self-talk to flood the mind – we are, after all, human (Wulf et al. 2010).

> Athletes in every sport will from time to time lose focus, become self-con-scious, have self-doubts to contend with and worry about things. . . . Emotions with strong physical components are the worst because they have what's called an attractor field – an energy field that can be quite intense and can affect the senses such as sight, hearing, touch, smell and taste. (Walker 2011, para. 1)

This debilitating shift of attention can occur to performers of any challeng-ing discipline. Gary Leffew, a stunt coordinator and rodeo rider, shared in an interview on NPR's *Fresh Air* that "Every time I look back . . . and a wreck happened . . . I was in a conscious thought process" (quoted in Wulf 2007, 21). Nicholas Le Riche, artistic director of the Royal Swedish Ballet, describes the same experience in performance, when interviewed for the Prix de Lausanne,

> It's terrible when you are on stage and when you start to struggle, then you start to question yourself and so you are not anymore in the mo-ment, because you are just looping in your head 'OK, I'm *not* going to

Attention and Focus in Practice

GIVE ME A CLEAR VISION!

Sorella Englund, international coach and ballet master, former principal dancer of The Royal Danish Ballet

If there is information coming from the outside all the time, from your teacher, your coach, your ballet master, there is no time to get *in* to yourself – and *you* are the one who is going to go out there, the one communicating what you have in your heart. It's so important to give dancers keys to trust their own 'voice'.

A new story ballet often *starts* with the drama and the relationship and then the physical demands take over. So, the story and intentions can get lost as we focus on perfecting. Dancers get physical information right up until the curtain goes – it's too much. We need time to explore 'What are we actually *saying* with this step?' So often dancers simply don't know where to focus.

I worked very intensely once with a dancer on the physicality, the drama, the passion of the role and then just before 'curtain up' on the premier, she spontaneously said 'Give me a vision!' No time to think, I just trusted what came out. I said 'freedom'. Before every performance she came to me, 'So what's for tonight?' and I suggested 'breathing the music', 'generosity' or 'sharing your vision'. I could see the focus helped her. All the corrections are *in there*; you don't need to think about them just before you perform. Follow a clear vision and let the music carry you.

We aim for the perfect all the time and that's fine to aim for something that makes us grow, but nobody *is* perfect. As long as we are human beings, we are not perfect and will never be. We need another image to go deeper, to be more honest, to dare to be true to ourselves and to the role we are developing. I think the word developing would be very good to take instead of perfecting. This 'perfect' business is killing the art.

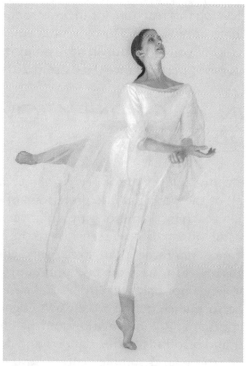

Figure 8.2   Dancer Kailey using the single cue word 'freedom'.

do this', 'Ahhgg, I have done it!', and it's completely wrong. (Prix de Lausanne 2020)

Developing the ability to reset the mind when the downward spiral of self-talk interrupts or to empty the mind of self-judgement with a 'goldfish brain' image when things don't go quite as planned and to avoid a 'wreck' is perhaps *the* most significant high-performance skill.

Becoming aware of the downward spiral of self-evaluation and self-talk as it starts during performance is a significant first step. As soon as you recognize the process, a quick recovery tip to reset the mind is to take the attention back to the breath, to expanding and making space for the in-coming breath and energy, and '. . . in one nanosecond, you bring mind and body together' (Watson 2019, attention and focus in practice, chapter 5). Allow the flow of the breath through and beyond the confines of your movement to dispel the increased muscular tension. Suspend for an instant with the sense of fullness, and as you turn the breathing wave around, power-out and re-place your planned attentional focus cue word or image on the sustained out-breath to reset the mind. If it is possible within the choreography, attend to the expanding and thorough emptying of the breath for a few cycles until your attention is back onto the effect of your movement and your sequence of chosen cues. Just like any aspect of technical performance, this recovery action becomes reflexive with practice. There is no need to wait for a performance emergency to develop this reaction. It can be introduced as an attentional tool into class, training or rehearsal. The more that you can implement this attention to the process of your attention in day-to-day dance practice, the less you will need recourse in performance (Hedstrom 2014).

ON A JOURNEY TOWARDS THE PRESENT

The cumulative effect of being open to attend to the process of attention; to all of the potential interpretations of external attentional focus in training, in teaching, in performing; to observe our intentions, our language, our transmission; to become sensitive to the nature and ceaseless flow of energy; to dance *with* rather than force *against* the nature of its universal movement opens the pathway to our own optimum growth and potential. As dancers we experience not only greater physical ease and increased energy and stamina in performance but also the freed cognitive reserve for enhanced recall of multidisciplinary information and heightened multisensory perception to hear and respond to other dancers and live musicians. The findings, theories, explorations and complementary strategies shared in this book provide a holistic support for the physical demands of Western dance technique that at the same time enable autonomy, enhancing capacities for individual communication and interpretation and provide freedom for artistry.

We are all deeply individual and must find our own learning paths, discover our own movement and perceptual patterns and find solutions to the challenges that *we* will face individually according to Oliver Sacks in his book *On the Move* (quoted in Watson 2017). However, I draw inspiration not from what divides us and makes us different, but rather from the elements that we share collectively, the elements that unite us all as dancers. We are all subject to the laws and the physics of the universe, and our dance is connected to the massive movement of the elements as we surf the continuum of energy. We must all manage the continual need for optimum breath drawn from a shared field of oxygen. We are inexorably bound by this simple binary action of expanding or contracting that is our movement and by the contrasting states of either receiving or giving, of replenishing or expending, of calm or action, of yin or yang. As human beings we distinguish ourselves from other beings by the ability to make conscious choices and to choose our response to a given stimulus. In any instant, we have the possibility to choose to bring our attention to this present moment at will – to consciously choose to shift the focus of our attention. Thank you for suspending your disbelief as we explored this frontier behind the eye. Let these uniting, universal elements inspire your explorations and let this opening become your daily practice of self-creation and your pathway to quantum change.

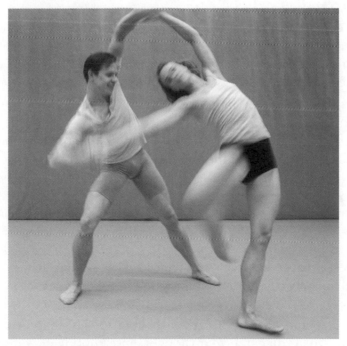

Figure 8.3   Dancers Tehri and Ben with attention 100 per cent in the moment.

It may feel as if we have done nothing, only given a little time and space of attention . . . some hairline-narrow crack opens . . . and there art, there beauty is. (Watson 2017, 142)

REFLECTION PROMPTS

Looking back through your reflective journal at our explorations, brainstorming and activities, what are the highlights or elements that most speak to you at this moment? Are there three or four that jump off the page and attract your attention? Are you already implementing some of them in your dance practice? Take those three or four as your first personal practice goals for development. Change will happen with least resistance when you start with what *attracts* and *brings you energy.*

- At the beginning, in chapter 1, you spontaneously answered the four questions from the professional dancer's attentional focus survey. Now that we have taken our journey together through external attentional focus, brainstormed potential external focus types and words, looked at supportive language and positively formulating information and optimal cueing, take a look at your original answers. Would you answer any of them differently today? Here are the questions again: *What do you focus on, imagine or think when preparing and executing a balance in fifth? A balance in arabesque? A pirouette en dehors? A grand jeté en avant?* Take a moment to draft your ideal self-cues or teaching cues for those four movements. Keep them close to hand in your journal and see if you can consciously implement this ideal wording the next time you take those movements in class. Your cues will naturally evolve as you discover what resonates best for you or works best for a particular group.

- In chapter 2, we asked ourselves about our habitual control approach in dance. Look back at the potential external focus types listed in figure 2.3. Have you explored other external focus types since we began? Note down the other EF types that you have added to your repertoire. We estimated our typical ratio of IF to EF (self-cues or teaching instructions and feedback). What was your score at the beginning of the book? We suggested ratios of perhaps 70:30, 50:50 or already 40:60. Would you say that ratio has already shifted? Give yourself a new score today and acknowledge your own progress in that short time.

- In class, start to practice the simple recovery technique of refocusing the attention on the breath discussed in this chapter to reset the mind when you catch your thoughts interrupting or wandering from your chosen image or cue. If you are a teacher, decide to teach it to students as a tool to reset their mind when self-related thoughts and the temptation for body-part adjustment takes over. In exploration 5.5, you gave yourself a score on a scale of 1 to 10 for your ability to reset your mind (table 5.2). How successfully do you feel you are you able to put thoughts to one side and reset your chosen attentional foci today? Once you start to practice mind reset, observe the process of your attention in class again and rate your ability, on a scale of 10, to reset your chosen attentional foci. How does today compare with the first rating you gave yourself?

EXPLORATION 8.1 – THE ULTIMATE EXTERNAL ATTENTIONAL FOCUS – CREATE A PERSONAL MISSION STATEMENT

We are on our own learning journey of developing awareness and observation, of defamiliarization with our habitual ways of approaching movement and of opening to our greatest potential. To guide your further explorations, you might like to create a personal, higher, external attentional focus that acts as an optimal high-performance cue aligning your actions and choices and supporting your performance, not only in dance but also in all aspects of your life. Complement your reflective tools by creating your own personal mission statement. You do not need to share it with anyone else; what's important is that it resonates with and inspires *you*.

Take a prominent page in your journal and write the following three headers – leaving plenty of space for writing around.

- To . . .
- With . . .
- Through my . . .

On a fresh page, take a few moments to brainstorm the following three questions, answering as spontaneously as possible:

1. Why do you dance? What is it that you would most like to bring to dance, to your teaching, to the dance world or to the public?

2. Think of a person that you most admire (this could be a family member, a friend, a colleague, a public person or even a fictional character). List their qualities, characteristics and attributes that you most admire. (Are they patient? Generous? Confident? Articulate? Fair?)

3. What are the areas or elements of your work you most enjoy? Or future areas of work you would most enjoy? Areas where you perhaps feel you can make a difference?

Your answers to number one go on the first line, your answers to number two on the second line, and your answers to number three go on the last line. It might take a little creative crafting and editing until you feel happy with your statement, until you have something that looks like this:

(continued)

EXPLORATION 8.1 *(continued)*

- To . . . *share my joy and bring healing and wisdom to dance*
- With . . . *consistency, clarity, energy and grace*
- Through my . . . *writing, my teaching and my lecturing*

It's not important that you are doing or manifesting all those things right now – it's a road map. Once you like the way it reads, refer to your mission statement as often as you can or use it as a kind of guiding mantra or affirmation. Your mission statement is not set in stone; it simply reflects where you would like to go to on your journey today. Revisit it regularly to reshape and hone it, perhaps a couple of times a year, and allow it to evolve as you answer spontaneously the same questions. At first you may find your answers and your statement oscillate wildly and change every six months as you find your way. However, eventually, as you hone in on your direction, you'll find it becomes more stable and refined with each maturation. Just as in dance, your higher, external attentional focus enables power and potential energy flow, releasing cognitive reserve for heightened multisensory perception and communication. Enjoy your explorations – enjoy the journey!

To share my joy and bring healing and wisdom to dance with consistency, clarity, energy and grace through my writing, my teaching and my lecturing.

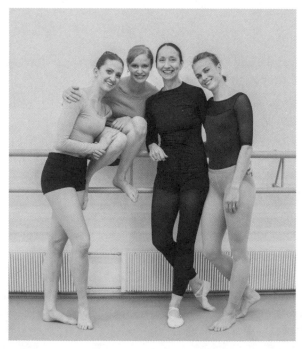

Figure 8.4   Sharing the joy of dance. (Kailey, Emmi, Clare and Tehri)

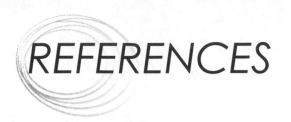

REFERENCES

Foreword

Krugman, Paul. 2020. "How Zombies Ate the G.O.P.'s Soul." *New York Times*, February 3, 2020. Accessed June 16, 2020. https://www.nytimes.com/2020/02/03/opinion/republican-party-trump.html?searchResultPosition=1

Lewthwaite, Rebecca, and Gabriele Wulf. 2010. "Grand Challenge for Movement Science and Sport Psychology: Embracing the Social-Cognitive–Affective–Motor Nature of Motor Behavior." *Frontiers in Psychology* 1: 42. www.ncbi.nlm.nih.gov/pmc/articles/PMC3153760

Wulf, Gabriele. 2013. "Attentional Focus and Motor Learning: A Review of 15 Years." *International Review of Sport and Exercise Psychology* 6: 77-104.

Wulf, Gabriele, Markus Höß, and Wolfgang Prinz. 1998. "Instructions for Motor Learning: Differential Effects of Internal Versus External Focus of Attention." *Journal of Motor Behavior* 30(2): 169-179.

Wulf, Gabriele, and Rebecca Lewthwaite. 2016. "Optimizing Performance Through Intrinsic Motivation and Attention for Learning: The OPTIMAL Theory of Motor Learning." *Psychonomic Bulletin & Review* 23: 1382-1414.

Preface

Chua, Lee-Kuen, Gabriele Wulf, and Rebecca Lewthwaite. 2018. "Onward and Upward: Optimizing Motor Performance." *Human Movement Science* 60: 107-114.

Guss-West, Clare, and Gabriele Wulf. 2016. "Attentional Focus in Classical Ballet: A Survey of Professional Dancers." *Journal of Dance Medicine & Science* 20(1): 23-29.

Myss, Caroline. 2017. "Choices That Can Change Your Life." TEDxFindhornSalon. Filmed April 2017. Video, 1:23. hwww.youtube.com/watch?v=-KysuBl2m_w

Watson, Gay. 2017. *Attention Beyond Mindfulness*. London: Reaktion Books.

Wulf, Gabriele. 2013. "Attentional Focus and Motor Learning: A Review of 15 Years." *International Review of Sport and Exercise Psychology* 6: 77-104.

Wulf, Gabriele. 2015. "An External Focus of Attention Is a Condition *Sine Qua Non* for Athletes: A Response to Carson, Collins, and Toner." *Journal of Sports Science* 34(13): 1293-1295. http://dx.doi.org/10.1080/02640414.2015.1136746

Wulf, Gabriele, and Rebecca Lewthwaite. 2016. "Optimizing Performance Through Intrinsic Motivation and Attention for Learning: The OPTIMAL Theory of Motor Learning." *Psychonomic Bulletin & Review* 23: 1382-1414.

Chapter 1

Cohn, Patrick. 2019. "Federer's Mental Game and Thinking Ahead." *Sports Psychology Tennis*, April 11, 2019. www.sportspsychologytennis.com/federers-mental-game-and-thinking-ahead

Guss-West, Clare, and Gabriele Wulf. 2016. "Attentional Focus in Classical Ballet: A Survey of Professional Dancers." *Journal of Dance Medicine & Science* 20(1): 23-29.

Hampson, Christopher. 2019. Personal interview. CEO and artistic director, Scottish Ballet, choreographer, dance educator, former soloist English National Ballet, July 1, 2019.

James, William. 1890. *The Principles of Psychology*. Cited in "William James Quotes." Brainy Quote. Last updated May 17, 2019. www.brainyquote.com/quotes/william_james_108497

Jäncke, Lutz. n.d. "Emotions Are the Glue Holding Our Travel Memories Together." *Moments That Last*. Accessed November 1, 2019. www.moments-that-last.com/en/article/67

Karin, Janet, and Sanna M. Nordin-Bates. 2019. "Enhancing Creativity and Managing Perfectionism in Dancers Through Implicit Learning and Sensori-Kinetic Imagery." *Journal of Dance Education*, April 30, 2019: 1-11. https://doi.org/10.1080/15290824.2018.1532572

Mackrell, Judith. 2009. "Zen and the Art of Dance." *The Guardian*, October 13, 2009. www.theguardian.com/stage/2009/oct/13/wayne-mcgregor-interview

McWilliams, Andrew. 2019. Personal interview. MBBS MRCPsych; specialist registrar in child and adolescent psychiatry; clinical research fellow: Great Ormond Street Hospital; Metacognition Lab, University College London; Psychological Medicine, King's College, July 11, 2019.

M.S., Pam N. 2013. "Focus." *Psychology Dictionary*. https://psychologydictionary.org/focus

Poikonen, Hanna. 2019. Personal interview. Neuroscientist, founder and director, WiseMotion Community, dance educator, dancer, postdoctoral researcher at the Institute of Learning Sciences and Higher Education, ETH Zurich, Switzerland, November 4, 2019.

Porter, Jared, Will Wu, and Julie Partridge. 2010. "Focus of Attention and Verbal Instructions: Strategies of Elite Track and Field Coaches and Athletes." *Sport Science Review* 19: 199-211.

Powers, Richard. 2010. "Use It or Lose It: Dancing Makes You Smarter, Longer." *Social Dance*, July 30, 2010. https://socialdance.stanford.edu/syllabi/smarter.htm

Retter, Greg. 2016. "Royal Commission." *Frontline, The Physiotherapy Magazine for CSP Members*, December 7, 2016. www.csp.org.uk/system/files/frontline_dec7_2016.pdf

Retter, Greg. 2019. Personal communication. Head of performance services, Team GB, former director of health care, The Royal Ballet, November 18, 2019.

Solway, Diane. 2007. "Learning to Dance, One Chunk at a Time." *New York Times*, May 27. www.nytimes.com/2007/05/27/arts/dance/27solw.html

Stoate, Isabelle, and Gabriele Wulf. 2011. "Does the Attentional Focus Adopted by Swimmers Affect Their Performance?" *International Journal of Sport Science & Coaching* 6: 99-108.

Study.com. n.d. "Attention as Part of Cognitive Development: Definition and Process." Human Growth and Development, Psychology Courses 6, Lesson 1. Accessed October 17, 2019. https://study.com/academy/lesson/attention-as-part-of-cognitive-development-definition-process.html

Taylor, Jim, and Elena Estanol. 2015. *Dance Psychology for Artistic and Performance Excellence*. Champaign, IL: Human Kinetics.

Thomson, Candice. 2018. "Why Do Some of the Most Talented Dancers Never 'Make It'?" *Dance Magazine*, August 6, 2018. www.dancemagazine.com/becoming-professional-dancer-2592408926.html

Watson, Gay. 2017. *Attention Beyond Mindfulness*. London: Reaktion Books.

Watson, Gay. n.d. "Attention." Text of a presentation given July 10, 2010, at the Institute of Oriental Philosophy, Taplow Manor. Accessed October 15, 2019. www.gaywatson.com/Attention.html

Wulf, Gabriele. 2007. *Attention and Motor Skill Learning*. Champaign, IL: Human Kinetics.

Wulf, Gabriele. 2013. "Attentional Focus and Motor Learning: A Review of 15 Years." *International Review of Sport and Exercise Psychology* 6: 77-104.

Wulf, Gabriele, and Wolfgang Prinz. 2001. "Directing Attention to Movement Effects Enhances Learning: A Review." *Psychonomic Bulletin & Review* 8(4): 648-660. https://link.springer.com/article/10.3758/BF03196201

Chapter 2

Abdollahipour, Reza, Gabriele Wulf, Rudolf Psotta, and Miriam Palomo Nieto. 2014. "Performance of Gymnastics Skills Benefits From an External Focus of Attention." *Journal of Sports Sciences* 33: 1807-1813.

Australian Ballet. 2018. "Ballet Anatomy: Hands." Last modified May 28, 2018. https://australianballet.com.au/tv/ballet-anatomy-hands

Dea, Greg. n.d. "Feedback and Cueing Part 2 – Reliable Strategies." On Target Publications. Accessed April 14, 2020. www.otpbooks.com/greg-dea-feedback-and-cueing-2

Eightyeightdays. 2018. "Implicit Motor learning - External Focus." Eight-Eight Days. Last modified April 30, 2018. https://eightyeightdays.com/2018/04/30/implicit-motor-learning-external-focus

Franklin, Eric. 1996. *Dance Imagery for Technique and Performance*. Champaign, IL: Human Kinetics.

Freudenheim, Andrea M., Gabriele Wulf, Fabricio Madureira, and Umberto C. Corrêa. 2010. "An External Focus of Attention Results in Greater Swimming Speed." *International Journal of Sports Science & Coaching* 5: 533-542.

Guss-West, Clare, and Gabriele Wulf. 2016. "Attentional Focus in Classical Ballet: A Survey of Professional Dancers." *Journal of Dance Medicine & Science* 20(1): 23-29.

Jarrett, Christian. 2015. "Want to Learn a New Skill Effectively? Stop Thinking About Yourself!" *Research Digest, The British Psychological Society*. Last modified February 9, 2015. https://digest.bps.org.uk/2015/02/09/want-to-learn-a-new-skill-more-effectively-stop-thinking-about-yourself

Kaba, Kailey. 2019. Personal interview. Professional ballet dancer, Finnish National Ballet; soloist, Ballett am Rhein; graduate of Canada's National Ballet School, July 9, 2019.

Karin, Janet, and Sanna M. Nordin-Bates. 2019. "Enhancing Creativity and Managing Perfectionism in Dancers Through Implicit Learning and Sensori-Kinetic Imagery." *Journal of Dance Education* (20)1: 1-11. https://doi.org/10.1080/15290824.2018.1532572

Kuhn, Yves-Alain, Martin Keller, Jan Ruffieux, and Wolfgang Taube. 2016. "Adopting an External Focus of Attention Alters Intracortical Inhibition Within the Primary Motor Cortex." *Acta Physiologica* 220(2): 289-299. https://doi.org/10.1111/apha.12807

Lawrence, Gavin P., Jana Virian, Samuel J. Oliver, and Victoria M. Gottwald. 2019. "Let's Go Surfing Now, Everybody's Learning How; Attentional Strategies on Expert and Novice Surfing Performance Under Both Practice and Competition Conditions." *European Journal of Sport Science* 20(2): 229-239. https://doi.org/10.1080/17461391.20 19.1626489

Lohse, Keith R., and David E. Sherwood. 2011. "Defining the Focus of Attention: Effects of Attention on Perceived Exertion and Fatigue." *Frontiers in Psychology* 2 (Article 332). https://doi.org/10.3389/fpsyg.2011.00332

Lohse, Keith R., David E. Sherwood, and Alice F. Healy. 2011. "Neuromuscular Effects of Shifting the Focus of Attention in a Simple Force Production Task." *Journal of Motor Behavior* 43: 173-184.

Marchant, David C., Peter J. Clough, Martin Crawshaw, and Andrew Levy. 2009. "Novice Motor Skill Performance and Task Experience Is Influenced by Attentional Focus Instructions and Instruction Preferences." *International Journal of Sport and Exercise Psychology* 7: 488-502.

Masters, Richard. 2014. "Motor Learning (Conscious and Non-Conscious) in Sport and Other Activities." UCD School of Psychology (University College Dublin, Ireland), Distinguished Scholar Public Lecture Filmed April 23, 2014. Last modified April 29, 2014. www.youtube.com/watch?v=jif6TMe_DcY

McNevin, Nancy H., Charles H. Shea, and Gabriele Wulf. 2003. "Increasing the Distance of an External Focus of Attention Enhances Learning." *Psychological Research* 67: 22-29.

McPherson, Gary E., and Barry J. Zimmerman. 2011. "Self-Regulation of Musical Learning: A Social Cognitive Perspective on Developing Performance Skills." In *MENC Handbook of Research on Music Learning. Volume 2: Applications*, edited by R. Colwell, and P.R. Webster (Eds.), 130-175. New York, NY: Oxford University Press.

McWilliams, Andrew. 2019. Personal interview. MBBS MRCPsych; specialist registrar in child and adolescent psychiatry, clinical research fellow: Great Ormond Street Hospital; Metacognition Lab, University College London; Psychological Medicine, King's College, July 11, 2019.

Mornell, Adina, and Gabriele Wulf. 2018. "Adopting an External Focus of Attention Enhances Musical Performance." *Journal of Research in Music Education* 66(4): 002242941880157. https://doi.org/10.1177/0022429418801573

Nordin, Sanna M., and Jennifer Cumming. 2006. "The Development of Imagery in Dance Part II: Quantitative Findings From a Mixed Sample of Dancers." *Journal of Dance Medicine and Science* 10(1/2): 28-34.

Nordin, Sanna M., and Jennifer Cumming. 2007. "Where, When, and How: A Quantitative Account of Dance Imagery." *Research Quarterly for Exercise and Sport* 78(4): 390-395.

Pavlik, Katherine, and Sanna Nordin-Bates. 2016. "Imagery in Dance: A Literature Review." *Journal of Dance Medicine & Science* 20: 51-63.

Pidgeon, Laura M., Madeleine Grealy, Alex H.B. Duffy, Laura Hay, Chris McTeague, Tijana Vuletic, Damien Coyle, and Sam J. Gilbert. 2016. "Functional Neuroimaging of Visual Creativity: A Systematic Review and Meta-Analysis." First published August 11, 2016. https://onlinelibrary.wiley.com/doi/full/10.1002/brb3.540

Porter, Jared M., Will W. Wu, and Julie A. Partridge. 2010. "Focus of Attention and Verbal Instructions: Strategies of Elite Track and Field Coaches and Athletes." *Sport Science Review* 19: 199-211.

Retter, Greg. 2019. Personal communication. Head of performance services, Team GB, former director of health care, The Royal Ballet, November 18, 2019.

Weiss, Stephen M., Arthur S. Reber, and David R. Owen. 2008. "The Locus of Focus: The Effect of Switching From a Preferred to a Non-Preferred Focus of Attention." *Journal of Sports Sciences* 26: 1049-1057.

Wulf, Gabriele. 2007. *Attention and Motor Skill Learning.* Champaign, IL: Human Kinetics.

Wulf, Gabriele. 2013. "Attentional Focus and Motor Learning: A Review of 15 Years." *International Review of Sport and Exercise Psychology* 6: 77-104.

Wulf, Gabriele, and Janet S. Dufek. 2009. "Increased Jump Height With an External Attentional Focus Is Due to Augmented Force Production." *Journal of Motor Behavior* 41: 401-409.

Wulf, Gabriele, Janet S. Dufek, Leonardo Lozano, and Christina Pettigrew. 2010. "Increased Jump Height and Reduced EMG Activity With an External Focus of Attention." *Human Movement Science* 29: 440-448. https://doi.org/10.1016/j.humov.2009.11.008

Wulf, Gabriele, Nancy H. McNevin, and Charles H. Shea. 2001. "The Automaticity of Complex Motor Skill Learning as a Function of Attentional Focus." *Quarterly Journal of Experimental Psychology* 54A: 1143-1154.

Wulf, Gabriele, Charles H. Shea, and Jin-Hoon Park. 2001. "Attention and Motor Learning: Preferences for and Advantages of an External Focus." *Research Quarterly for Exercise and Sport* 72: 335-344.

Wulf, Gabriele, Thomas Töllner, and Charles H. Shea. 2007. "Attentional Focus Effects as a Function of Task Difficulty." *Research Quarterly for Exercise and Sport* 78(3): 257. https://doi.org/10.1080/02701367.2007.10599423

Zachry, Tiffany L. 2005. "Effects of Attentional Focus on Kinematics and Muscle Activation Patterns as a Function of Expertise." Unpublished master's thesis, University of Nevada, Las Vegas. Accessed April 13, 2020. https://digitalscholarship.unlv.edu/cgi/viewcontent.cgi?article=2861&context=rtds

Chapter 3

Bennett, Bija. 1993. *Breathing Into Life.* Minnesota: Hazelden Education Materials.

Brecher, Paul. 2001. *Secrets of Energy Work.* London: Dorling Kindersley.

Brennen, Barbara Ann. 1988. *Hands of Light; A Guide to Healing Through the Human Energy Field.* New York: Bantam Books.

Chai, Raymond. 2019. Personal interview. Lecturer in dance, The Place, London, choreographer, ballet master and guest teacher, former professional dancer, National Ballet of Portugal, The Royal Shakespeare Company, July 31, 2019.

Collette, David. 2019. "Kung Fu Tea (Everything You Need to Know)," Liquid Mageco. Last updated September 3, 2019. www.liquidimageco.com/kung-fu-tea

Dirlam Ching, Elise, and Kaleo Ching. 2007. *Chi and Creativity: Vital Energy and Your Inner Artist*. Vermont: Blue Snake Books.

Fraser, Jack. 2017. "How the Human Body Creates Electromagnetic Fields." *Forbes*. Last updated November 3, 2017. www.forbes.com/sites/quora/2017/11/03/how-the-human-body-creates-electromagnetic-fields/#68084f0d56ea

Jahnke, Roger. 2002. *The Healing Promise of Qi*. New York: Contemporary Books.

Kam Chuen, Lam. 1991. *The Way of Energy*. London: Gaia Books.

Kam Chuen, Lam. 2003. *The Way of Power*. Champaign, IL: Human Kinetics.

Lopez Rio, Agnès. 2019. Personal interview. Professional dancer, formerly Compañia Nacional de Danza, Company Wayne McGregor, artistic consultant, choreographer, dance educator Conservatorio Superior de Danza de Madrid, María de Ávila, July 24, 2019.

Martin, Meredith. 2015. "Mirror Reflections: Louis XIV, Phra Narai, and the Material Culture of Kingship." Association of Art Historians. 652-667. Academia.edu. Accessed April 14, 2020. www.academia.edu/23498704/Mirror_Reflections_Louis_XIV_Phra_Narai_and_the_Material_Culture_of_Kingship

McTaggart, Lynne. 2003. *The Field*. London: Harper Collins.

Mornell, Adina, and Gabriele Wulf. 2019. "Adopting an External Focus of Attention Enhances Musical Performance." *Journal of Research in Music Education* 66(4): 375-391.

Quian, Rene. 2017. *The MSCP (The Mental Screen Conditioning Process-I-Routine) Principle*. New York: Page Publishing.

Rodell, Scott. 2017. "Energy Centers in the Body: Culture and History Overlap." T'ai Chi Basics. Last updated April 1, 2017. https://taichibasics.com/energy-centers-in-the-body-affid341502

Sundermier, Ali. 2016. "99.9999999% of Your Body Is Empty Space." *Science Alert, Business Insider*. Last updated September 23, 2016. www.sciencealert.com/99-9999999-of-your-body-is-empty-space

Thackeray, William Makepeace. n.d. "King Canute." All Poetry. Accessed November 1, 2019. https://allpoetry.com/King-Canute

Taylor, Jim. 2015. "Concentration in Dance." Dr Jim Taylor. Last updated June 12, 2015. www.drjimtaylor.com/4.0/concentration-in-dance

Watson, Gay. 2017. *Attention Beyond Mindfulness*. London: Reaktion Books.

Watts, Dennis. n.d. "Energy of the Body." T'ai Chi Association of Australia. Accessed October 31, 2019. www.taichiaustralia.com/articles/Energy_of_the_body.htm

Wilkens, Andreas, Michael Jacobi, and Wolfram Schwenk. 2005. *Understanding Water – Developments From the Work of Theodor Schwenk*. Translated by David Auerbach and Jennifer Greene. Edinburgh: Floris Books.

Wulf, Gabriele. 2007. *Attention and Motor Skill Learning*. Champaign, IL: Human Kinetics.

Chapter 4

Flatow, Sheryl. n.d. "Sorella Englund: Defining Character." Boston Ballet. Accessed June 16, 2020. www.bostonballet.org/Home/BehindTheScenes/Sorella-Englund-Defining-Character.aspx

Freedman, Joshua. 2016. "Practicing Emotional Intelligence." Six Seconds eBook, 13. Accessed April 14, 2020. www.6seconds.org/?s=Practicing+emotional+intelligence+Pdf

Guss-West, Clare. 2014. "Holistic Ballet." In *The Song of The Body*, edited by Anne Hogan, 130-137. London: Royal Academy of Dance Enterprises Ltd.

Guss-West, Clare, and Gabriele Wulf. 2016. "Attentional Focus in Classical Ballet: A Survey of Professional Dancers." *Journal of Dance Medicine & Science* 20(1): 23-29.

Hopper, Luke S., Andries L. Weidemann, and Janet Karin. 2018. "The Inherent Movement Variability Underlying Classical Ballet Technique and the Expertise of a Dancer." *Research in Dance Education* 19(3): 229-239. https://doi.org/10.1080/14647893.2017.1420156

Lexico. 2017. "Arabesque." Lexico. Accessed September 19, 2019. www.lexico.com/en/definition/arabesque

Liponis, Mark. 2007. "Ultra Longevity." New York: Little, Brown and Co.

Martin, Paul. 2019. "Who Said 'The Whole Is Greater Than the Sum of the Parts'?" SE Scholar. Last modified June 6, 2019. http://se-scholar.com/se-blog/2017/6/23/who-said-the-whole-is-greater-than-the-sum-of-the-parts

Myss, Caroline. 1998. *Anatomy of the Spirit*. London: Bantam Books.

National Ballet of Canada. 2019. "William Forsythe: Inside the Studio." The National Ballet of Canada video. Posted May 3, 2019. https://national.ballet.ca/Productions/2018-19-Season/Physical-Thinking

Quian, Rene. 2017. *The MSCP (The Mental Screen Conditioning Process-I-Routine) Principle*. New York: Page Publishing.

Quote investigator. n.d. Accessed April 14, 2020. https://quoteinvestigator.com/2016/04/25/get/#note-13559-1

Ryman, Rhonda (ed.). 2008. *The Foundations of Classical Ballet Technique*. London: The Royal Academy of Dance, Enterprises.

Saland, Stephanie. 2019. Personal interview. Dance educator and coach, former principal dancer, New York City Ballet, March 8, 2019.

Torres, Javier. 2019. Personal interview. International ballet teacher, coach, choreographer, former dancer with the Finnish National Ballet, June 11, 2019.

Watson, Gay. 2017. *Attention Beyond Mindfulness*. London: Reaktion Books.

Watts, Dennis. n.d. "Energy of the Body." T'ai Chi Association of Australia. Accessed October 31, 2019. www.taichiaustralia.com/articles/Energy_of_the_body.htm

West, Clare. 1997. *The Energy Source: Simple Daily Exercise for Mind and Body Vitality*. London: Prion Books.

Wright, Janet. 2001. *Reflexology and Acupressure*. London: Hamlyn.

Wulf, Gabriele. 2013. "Attentional Focus and Motor Learning: A Review of 15 Years." *International Review of Sport and Exercise Psychology* 6: 77-104.

Chapter 5

Bradberry, Travis. 2014. "How (and Why) to Stay Positive." Rice University Educational Blog. Accessed July 22, 2019. http://blogs.rice.edu

Bradberry, Travis. 2017. "The Power of Emotional Intelligence." TEDx Talks University of California, August 3, 2017. www.youtube.com/watch?v=auXNnTmhHsk

Brecher, Paul. 2001. *Secrets of Energy Work*. London: Dorling Kindersley.

Dalleck, Lance C. n.d. "The Science of Post-Exercise Recovery." American Council on Exercise. Ace Fitness. Accessed April 15, 2020. https://acewebcontent.azureedge.net/SAP-Reports/Post-Exercise_Recovery_SAP_Reports.pdf

Foong, Albert. n.d. "How to Develop Visualization Skill." Litemind. Accessed April 15, 2020. https://litemind.com/how-to-develop-visualization-skill

Franklin, Eric. 2014. *Dance Imagery for Technique and Performance*. Champaign, IL: Human Kinetics.

Hani, Julie. 2017. "The Neuroscience of Behaviour Change." Health Transformer. Last modified August 8, 2017. https://healthtransformer.co/the-neuroscience-of-behavior-change-bcb567fa83c1

Harari, Dana, Brian W. Swider, Laurens B. Steed, and Amy P. Breidenthal. 2018. "Is Perfect Good? A Meta-Analysis of Perfectionism in the Workplace." *Journal of Applied Psychology* 103(10): 1121-1144.

Jahnke, Roger. 2002. *The Healing Promise of Qi*. New York: Contemporary Books.

Kaba, Kailey. 2019. Personal interview. Professional ballet dancer, Finnish National Ballet; soloist, Ballett am Rhein; graduate of Canada's National Ballet School, July 9, 2019.

Kam Chuen, Lam. 2003. *The Way of Power*. Champaign, IL: Human Kinetics.

Lee, Abby. 2016. "Small Circulation of Chi." Qi Gong Melbourne. Last modified February 5, 2016. https://qigongmelbourne.com.au/resources/student-resources/zhan-zhung-2

McWilliams, Andrew. 2019. Personal interview. MBBS MRCPsych; specialist registrar in child and adolescent psychiatry, clinical research fellow: Great Ormond Street Hospital; Metacognition Lab, University College London; Psychological Medicine, King's College London, July 11, 2019.

MedicineNet. n.d. "The Sacrum . . . the Holy Bone." Accessed April 15, 2020. www.medicinenet.com/script/main/art.asp?articlekey=6970

Myss, Caroline. 1998. *Why People Don't Heal and How They Can*. London: Bantam Books.

Osho. n.d. "The Ultimate Alchemy, Vol. 2, Talk 1." Highlights of Oshos World. Accessed April 15, 2020. www.osho.com/highlights-of-oshos-world/osho-on-awareness-quotes

Paskevska, Anna. n.d. "On Zen, Flow, and Being in the Dance." Tall Skinny. Accessed April 15, 2020. www.tallskinny.com/anna/art1.html

Prath, Scott. 2019. "Conception Vessel." T'ai Chi Basics. Last modified March 1, 2019. https://taichibasics.com/conception-vessel

Quian, Rene. 2017. *The MSCP (The Mental Screen Conditioning Process-I-Routine) Principle*. New York: Page Publishing.

Ryman, Rhonda (ed.). 2008. *The Foundations of Classical Ballet Technique*. London: The Royal Academy of Dance, Enterprises Ltd.

Taylor, Jim. 2015. "Concentration in Dance." Dr Jim Taylor. Last modified June 12, 2015. www.drjimtaylor.com/4.0/concentration-in-dance

Watson, Gay. 2019. Personal interview. Lecturer, psychotherapist, writer, June 24, 2019.

Wulf, Gabriele. 2007. *Attention and Motor Skill Learning*. Champaign, IL: Human Kinetics.

Wulf, Gabriele, and Rebecca Lewthwaite. 2016. "Optimizing Performance Through Intrinsic Motivation and Attention for Learning: The OPTIMAL Theory of Motor Learning." *Psychonomic Bulletin & Review* 5: 1382-1414.

Zar, Rachel. 2018. "The Expert-Approved Training Plan for Time Off From Dance." *Dance Magazine*, June 1, 2018. www.dancemagazine.com/periodization-2569974392.html

Chapter 6

Abdollahipour, Reza, Gabriele Wulf, Rudolf Psotta, and Miriam Palomo Nieto. 2014. "Performance of Gymnastics Skills Benefits From an External Focus of Attention." *Journal of Sports Sciences* 33: 1807-1813.

Adams, A.J. 2009. "Seeing Is Believing – The Power of Visualization." *Psychology Today*. Last modified December 3, 2009. www.psychologytoday.com/intl/blog/flourish/200912/seeing-is-believing-the-power-visualization

Assandri, Eric P.J. 2019. "Is 'Touching' Essential When Teaching Ballet?" *Research in Dance Education* 20(2): 197-207. https://doi.org/10.1080/14647893.2019.1609435

Bannon, Fiona, and Duncan Holt. 2012. "Engaging With Touch: Transformative Learning in Dance." AusDance. Accessed April 23, 2020. https://ausdance.org.au/uploads/content/publications/2012-global-summit/dance-learning-rp/engaging-with-touch-transformative-learning-in-dance.pdf

Chai, Raymond. 2019. Personal interview. MA, lecturer in dance, The Place, London, choreographer, ballet master and guest teacher, former professional dancer, July 31, 2019.

Fitts, Paul. 1964. "Perceptual-Motor Skill Learning." In *Categories of Human Learning*, edited by A.W. Melton, pp. 243-285. New York: Academic Press.

Fleming, Neil D., and Christine Mills. 1992. "Not Another Inventory, Rather a Catalyst for Reflection." *To Improve the Academy* 11: 137-155.

Guss-West, Clare, and Gabriele Wulf. 2016. "Attentional Focus in Classical Ballet: A Survey of Professional Dancers," *Journal of Dance Medicine & Science* 20(1): 23-29.

Karin, Janet, and Sanna M. Nordin-Bates. 2019. "Enhancing Creativity and Managing Perfectionism in Dancers Through Implicit Learning and Sensori-Kinetic Imagery." *Journal of Dance Education* 20(1): 1-11. https://doi.org/10.1080/15290824.2018.1532572

Lambert, Craig. 2012. "Twilight of the Lecture." *Harvard Magazine*. March-April 2012. https://harvardmagazine.com/2012/03/twilight-of-the-lecture

Lyden, Jacki. 2009. "'Bye-Bye Birdie' Actor Finds It Odd to Have a Body." *NPR Weekend Edition*. October 3, 2009. www.npr.org/templates/story/story.php?storyId=113465178?storyId=113465178&t=1576764978246

Masters, Rich. 2014. "Motor Learning (Conscious and Non-Conscious) in Sport and Other Activities." UCD School of Psychology (University College Dublin, Ireland), Distinguished Scholar Public Lecture filmed April 23, 2014. Last modified April 29, 2014. www.youtube.com/watch?v=jif6TMe_DcY

Mazur, Eric. 2009. "Farewell, Lecture?" *Science* 323(5910): 50-51. https://doi.org/10.1126/science.1168927

Nordin, Sanna M., and Jennifer Cumming. 2007. "Where, When, and How: A Quantitative Account of Dance Imagery." *Research Quarterly of Exercise & Sport* 78(4): 390-395.

Nordin-Bates, Sanna M. 2019. Personal interview. PhD CPsychol FIADMS, senior lecturer, Swedish School of Sport and Health Sciences, Stockholm; chartered psychologist, British Psychological Society; Fellow of the International Association for Dance Medicine and Science, August 18, 2019.

Outevsky, David. 2013. "The Role of Touch as a Teaching and Learning Tool in Dance." *Journal of Emerging Dance Scholarship*. July 2013. www.jedsonline.net/wp-content/uploads/2013/07/THE-ROLE-OF-TOUCH-AS-A-TEACHING-AND.pdf

Pavlik, Katherine, and Sanna Nordin-Bates. 2016. "Imagery in Dance: A Literature Review." *Journal of Dance Medicine & Science* 20: 51-63.

Porter, Jared M., Will W. Wu, and Julie A. Partridge. 2010. "Focus of Attention and Verbal Instructions: Strategies of Elite Track and Field Coaches and Athletes." *Sport Science Review* 19: 199-211.

University of Iowa. 2006. "V.A.R.K." The Center for Teaching. Accessed April 23, 2020. https://teach.its.uiowa.edu/sites/teach.its.uiowa.edu/files/docs/docs/VARK_ed.pdf

Vark Learn. n.d. "The Vark Modalities." Vark Learn. Accessed April 23, 2020. https://vark-learn.com/introduction-to-vark/the-vark-modalities/?p=categories%20Fleming,%20N.%20D

Williamson, Marianne. 2004. *Everyday Grace*. New York: Riverhead Books.

Wulf, Gabriele. 2013. "Attentional Focus and Motor Learning: A Review of 15 Years." *International Review of Sport and Exercise Psychology* 6: 77-104.

Wulf, Gabriele. 2014. "Changing Patients Focus of Attention to Enhance Motor Performance and Learning." Doc Player. Presentation at APTA Combined Sections Meeting, Las Vegas, NV, 2014. Accessed April 23, 2020. https://docplayer.net/37280022-Changing-patients-focus-of-attention-to-enhance-motor-performance-and-learning.html

Wulf, Gabriele, Thomas Töllner, and Charles H. Shea. 2007. "Attentional Focus Effects as a Function of Task Difficulty." *Research Quarterly for Exercise and Sport* 78(3): 257-264. https://doi.org/10.1080/02701367.2007.10599423

Chapter 7

Boesch, Natalia. 2018. "Fouetté Turns: Secrets of the Cuban Method." *Pointe Magazine*, December 14, 2018. www.pointemagazine.com/fouette-turn-tricks-ballet-2623235430.html?rebelltitem=1#rebelltitem1

Chiviacowsky, Suzete, and Gabriele Wulf. 2007. "Feedback After Good Trials Enhances Learning." *Research Quarterly for Exercise and Sport* 78: 40-47.

Chiviacowsky, Suzete, Gabriele Wulf, Raquel Wally, and Thiago Borges. 2009. "Knowledge of Results After Good Trials Enhances Learning in Older Adults." *Research Quarterly for Exercise and Sport* 80: 663-668.

Chua, Lee-Kuen, Gabriele Wulf, and Rebecca Lewthwaite. 2018. "Onward and Upwards: Optimizing Motor Performance." *Human Movement Science* 60: 107-114.

Deci, Edward L., and Richard M. Ryan. 2000. "The 'What' and 'Why' of Goal Pursuits: Human Needs and the Self-Determination of Behavior." *Psychological Inquiry* 11: 227-268.

Ewell, Laura A., and Stefan Leutgeb. 2014. "Replay to Remember: A Boost From Dopamine." *Nature Neuroscience* 17: 1629-1631.

Hampson, Christopher. 2018. "Behaviour in the Ballet World." Scottish Ballet. March 5, 2018. www.scottishballet.co.uk/articles/behaviour-in-the-ballet-world

Hampson, Christopher. 2019. Personal interview. CEO and artistic director of the Scottish Ballet, choreographer, dance educator, former soloist of the English National Ballet, July 1, 2019.

Hooyman, Andrew, Gabriele Wulf, and Rebecca Lewthwaite. 2014. "Impacts of Autonomy-Supportive Versus Controlling Instructional Language on Motor Learning." *Human Movement Science* 36: 190-198.

Kokkonen, Timo. 2019. Personal interview. Dance educator at the Finnish National Ballet, former professional dancer. May 3, 2019.

Langer, Ellen J., and Judith Rodin. 1976. "The Effects of Choice and Enhanced Personal Responsibility for the Aged: A Field Experiment in an Institutional Setting." *Journal of Personality and Social Psychology* 34(2): 191-198.

Lewthwaite, Rebecca, Suzette Chiviacowsky, Ricardo Drews, and Gabriele Wulf. 2015. "Choose to Move: The Motivational Impact of Autonomy Support on Motor Learning." *Psychonomic Bulletin & Review* 22: 1383-1388.

Mosston, Muska, and Sara Ashworth. 1994. *Teaching Physical Education*. New York: Macmillan Publishing Co.

National Ballet of Canada. 2019. "William Forsythe: Inside the Studio." The National Ballet of Canada video. Posted May 3, 2019. https://national.ballet.ca/Productions/2018-19-Season/Physical-Thinking

Pennell, Kate Maria. 2017. "Living Without Limiting Your Potential: The Difference Between Expectation and Expectancy." *Medium*. June 5, 2017. https://medium.com/@KateMariaPennell/expectation-vs-expectancy-862c7e6ec184

Reeve, Johnmarshall, and Ching-Mei Tseng. 2011. "Cortisol Reactivity to a Teacher's Motivating Style: The Biology of Being Controlled Versus Supporting Autonomy." *Motivation and Emotion* 35: 63-74.

Saemi, Esmaeel, Gabriele Wulf, Ahmad Gohtbi Varzaneh, and Mehdi Zarghami. 2011. "Feedback After Good Versus Poor Trials Enhances Motor Learning in Children." *Revista Brasileira de Educação Fiscica e Esporte* 25: 673-681.

Stoate, Isabelle, and Gabriele Wulf. 2011. "Does the Attentional Focus of Swimmers Affect Their Performance?" *International Journal of Sports Science and Coaching* 6: 99-108.

Trempe, Maxime, Maxime Sabourin, and Luc Proteau. 2012. "Success Modulates Consolidation of a Visuomotor Adaptation Task." *Journal of Experimental Psychology: Learning Memory and Cognition* 38: 52-60.

Wulf, Gabriele, Suzete Chiviacowsky, and Priscila Cardozo. 2014. "Additive Benefits of Autonomy Support and Enhanced Expectancies for Motor Learning." *Human Movement Science* 37: 12-20.

Wulf, Gabriele, Suzete Chiviacowsky, and Rebecca Lewthwaite. 2012. "Altering Mind-Set Can Enhance Motor Learning in Older Adults." *Psychology and Aging* 27: 14-21.

Wulf, Gabriele, Suzete Chiviacowsky, Eduardo Schiller, and Luciana Toaldo Gentilini Avila. 2010. "Frequent External Focus Feedback Enhances Motor Learning." *Frontiers in Psychology* November 11, 1(190): 1-22.

Wulf, Gabriele, Heidi E. Freitas, and Richard D. Tandy. 2014. "Choosing to Exercise More: Small Choices Can Increase Exercise Engagement." *Psychology of Sport and Exercise* 15: 268-271.

Wulf, Gabriele, and Rebecca Lewthwaite. 2016. "Optimizing Performance Through Intrinsic Motivation and Attention for Learning: The OPTIMAL Theory of Motor Learning." *Psychonomic Bulletin & Review* 23: 1382-1414.

Wulf, Gabriele, Rebecca Lewthwaite, Priscila Cardozo, and Suzete Chiviacowsky. 2018. "Triple Play: Additive Contributions of Enhanced Expectancies, Autonomy Support and External Attentional Focus to Motor Learning." *Quarterly Journal of Experimental Psychology* 71(4): 824-831.

Chapter 8

Australian Ballet. 2018. "Ballet Anatomy: Eyes." Video posted June 14, 2018. https://australianballet.com.au/tv/ballet-anatomy-eyes

Benz, Adam, Nick Winkelman, Jared Porter, and Sophia Nimphius. 2016. "Coaching Instructions and Cues for Enhancing Sprint Performance." *Strength and Conditioning Journal* 38(1): 1-11.

Brigham Young University. n.d. "How to Give Better Feedback." Center for Teaching and Learning. Accessed April 21, 2020. https://ctl.byu.edu/tip/how-give-better-feedback

Chiviacowsky, Suzete, and Gabriele Wulf. 2002. "Self-Controlled Feedback: Does It Enhance Learning Because Performers Get Feedback When They Need It?" *Research Quarterly for Exercise and Sport* 73(4): 408-415.

Chiviacowsky, Suzete, and Gabriele Wulf. 2007. "Feedback After Good Trials Enhances Learning." *Research Quarterly for Exercise and Sport* 78: 40-47.

Chiviacowsky, Suzete, Gabriele Wulf, Raquel Wally, and Thiago Borges. 2009. "Knowledge of Results After Good Trials Enhances Learning in Older Adults." *Research Quarterly for Exercise and Sport* 80: 663-668.

Clark, Shannon. E., and Diane M. Ste-Marie. 2007. "The Impact of Self-as-a-Model Interventions on Children's Self-Regulation of Learning and Swimming Performance." *Journal of Sports Science* 25: 577-586.

Englund, Sorella. 2019. Personal interview. International coach and ballet master, permanent guest teacher National Ballet School, Canada, former principal dancer, The Royal Danish Ballet, educated Finnish National Opera Ballet School, August 5, 2019.

Glasstone, Richard. 1991. "Do Ballet Teachers Speak Too Much?" *The Dance Gazette* 208: 32-33.

Guss-West, Clare, and Gabriele Wulf. 2016. "Attentional Focus in Classical Ballet: A Survey of Professional Dancers." *Journal of Dance Medicine & Science* 20(1): 23-29.

Hanshaw, George. 2018. "Use Imagery and Self-Talk to Create an Immediate Reduction in Response Time." *Applied Sports Psychology*. March 8, 2018. Accessed April 20, 2020. https://appliedsportpsych.org/blog/2018/03/use-imagery-and-self-talk-to-create-an-immediate-reduction-in-response-time/

Hedstrom, Ryan. 2014. "Cue Statements: Staying Focused at Critical Times." *Applied Sports Psychology*. August 14, 2014. https://appliedsportpsych.org/blog/2014/08/cue-statements-staying-focused-at-critical-times

Kaba, Kailey. 2019. Personal interview. Professional ballet dancer, Finnish National Ballet; soloist, Ballett am Rhein; graduate of Canada's National Ballet School, July 9, 2019.

Karin, Janet, and Sanna M. Nordin-Bates. 2019. "Enhancing Creativity and Managing Perfectionism in Dancers Through Implicit Learning and Sensori-Kinetic Imagery." *Journal of Dance Education* 20(1): 1-11. https://doi.org/10.1080/15290824.2018.1532572

Lambert, Craig. 2012. "The Twilight of the Lecture." *Harvard Magazine*. March-April 2012. https://harvardmagazine.com/2012/03/twilight-of-the-lecture

LeBorgne, Wendy D., and Marci Daniels Rosenberg. 2021. *The Vocal Athlete*. 2nd ed. San Diego, CA: Plural Publishing.

Lexicon. n.d. "Definition of Feedback." Lexicon. Accessed April 20, 2020. https://www.lexico.com/en/definition/feedback

Meadows-Fernandez, Rochaun. 2017. "What Is Extrinsic Motivation and Is It Effective?" *Health Line*. September 25, 2017. www.healthline.com/health/extrinsic-motivation

Onne, Madeleine. 2019. Personal interview. Artistic director Finnish National Ballet, teacher, former soloist of Dallas Ballet and principal dancer of The Royal Swedish Ballet, July 10, 2019.

Osho. n.d. "The Book of Secrets." Talk #28. Osho Quotes on Awareness, Highlights of Osho's World. Accessed April 20, 2020. www.osho.com/highlights-of-oshos-world/osho-on-awareness-quotes

Poikonen, Hanna. 2020. Personal communication. Neuroscientist, founder and director Wise Motion Community, dance educator, dancer, postdoctoral researcher at the Institute of Learning Sciences and Higher Education, ETH Zurich, Switzerland, February 20, 2020.

Poirier Leroy, Olivier. n.d. "The Ridiculous Power of Performance Cues for Swimmers." Your Swim Book. www.yourswimlog.com/performance-cues

Prix de Lausanne. 2020. "Prix de Lausanne 2020 live interviews." Interviewed by Emma Sandall and Jason Beechey. Prix de Lausanne, Day 3 Afternoon. February 5, 2020. 1:00:12. Accessed April 20, 2020. www.youtube.com/watch?v=7y2ghWcYAj8&feature=share

Rathle, Karine. 2018. "I Stand Corrected! From Correction to Constructive Feedback." IADMS. Last modified June 4, 2018. www.iadms.org/blogpost/1177934/General?tag=motor+learning

Rist, Rachael. 2001. "Giving Feedback When Teaching." *Dancing Times Magazine*, February 2001.

Saemi, Esmaeel, Gabriele Wulf, Ahmad Gohtbi Varzaneh, and Mehdi Zarghami. 2011. "Feedback After Good Versus Poor Trials Enhances Motor Learning in Children." *Revista Brasileira de Educação Fisica e Esporte* 25: 673-681.

Thomson, Candice. 2018. "Why Do Some of The Most Talented Dancers Never 'Make It'?" *Dance Magazine*, August 6, 2018. www.dancemagazine.com/becoming-professional-dancer-2592408926.html

Walker, Stephen. 2011. "Recovery From Distractions Fast: The Thought Pattern Interrupt (TPI)." *Podium Sports Journal*, September 9, 2011. www.podiumsportsjournal.com/2011/09/09/the-thought-pattern-interrupt-tpi

Watson, Gay. 2017. *Attention Beyond Mindfulness*. London: Reaktion Books.

Watson, Gay. 2019. Personal interview. Lecturer, psychotherapist, writer, June 24, 2019.

Wegner, Daniel M., David J. Schneider, Samuel R. Carter, and Teri L. White. 1987. "Paradoxical Effects of Thoughts Suppression." *Journal of Personality and Social Psychology* 53: 5-13.

Wiggins, Grant. 2012. "Seven Keys to Effective Feedback." *Educational Leadership* 70(1): 10-16. www.ascd.org/publications/educational-leadership/sept12/vol70/num01/Seven-Keys-to-Effective-Feedback.aspx

Wulf, Gabriele. 2007. *Attention and Motor Skill Learning*. Champaign, IL: Human Kinetics.

Wulf, Gabriele. 2013. "Attentional Focus and Motor Learning: A Review of 15 Years." *International Review of Sport and Exercise Psychology* 6: 77-104.

Wulf, Gabriele, Suzete Chiviacowsky, Eduardo Schiller, and Luciana Toaldo Gentilini Ávila. 2010. "Frequent External-Focus Feedback Enhances Learning." *Frontiers in Psychology* 1(190): 1-7.

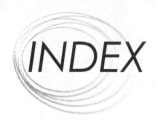

INDEX

Note: The italicized *f* and *t* following page numbers refer to figures and tables, respectively.

ABOUT THE AUTHOR

Clare Guss-West is a former professional dancer, choreographer, holistic health practitioner and author specialising in the integration of holistic health and dance.

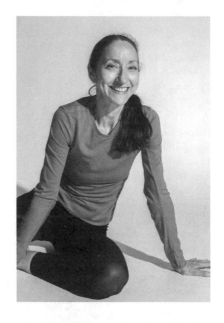

Clare's innovative work translates recent scientific research findings on attentional focus for direct application in professional, vocational and inclusive dance practice. Supported by her Eastern-movement practice, she provides mindful attention and focus strategies that harness mind, energy and effort to empower dancers, giving them the edge and the tools to enhance their own physical and mental performance and achieve their best. She shares this work with the dancers, teachers and health care teams of such companies and educational organisations as Finnish National Ballet and School, The Royal Ballet, Houston Ballet, Ballet de L'Opéra du Rhin, Opéra de Paris–Opéra Université, Dutch National Ballet Education, Pôle Supérieur de Danse Rosella Hightower and the Nureyev Foundation as well as the Royal Academy of Dance (RAD) international CPD program.

To facilitate inclusive dance practice, Clare adapts attentional focus theories as effective teaching tools to enable movement, promote creativity and restore well-being. She employs this approach in her Danse Senior projects at Konzert Theater Bern Dance Company and teaches it on the MAS Dance Science, Bern University, the University Diploma, 'Dance, Health & Aging', University Côte d'Azur and in RAD's CPD module Dance for Adults and Older Learners.

Trained as a classical and contemporary dancer and musician, Clare began choreographing with American composer Philip Glass and was resident choreographer and director at English National Opera. She has created productions for Lyric Opera of Chicago, Los Angeles Opera, Seattle Opera, San Francisco Opera and Ballet, Dutch National Opera and Ballet, Royal Opera House, BBC Proms and Opéra de Paris.

As cofounder and director of the Dance & Creative Wellness Foundation (launched with the support of Dutch National Ballet) and chair of the Dance for Health committee of the International Association for Dance Medicine & Science (IADMS), she is an international advocate of the well-being benefits of dance and its role in innovative preventative health.